# The Finest Cut

One Person's Experience With Transsexual Surgery

by

*Jean Churchill*

# TABLE OF CONTENTS


LET'S START AT THE VERY BEGINNING ........................ 2

COUNTDOWN TO SURGERY .......................................... 9

SURGERY AND THE HOSPITAL STAY ........................... 35

WHAT ACTUALLY HAPPENS DURING THIS
OPERATION? ............................................................... 37

RECUPERATION AT THE 'RESIDENCE' ......................... 56

RECUPERATION AT HOME .............................................. 96

FREQUENTLY ASKED QUESTIONS .............................. 108

WHERE DOES JEAN FEEL THAT SHE FITS IN ............. 112

# LET'S START AT THE VERY BEGINNING

Actually, let's not.  If you are reading this, you've probably also read any number of transsexual auto-biographies detailing the struggles that we deal with in recognizing and living our authentic identities.  My struggles were not much different from most of what you have already read.  So, instead, in this little memoir, I'm going to concentrate only on the circumstances shortly before and surrounding my sexual reassignment surgery (SRS), on some of my thoughts and feelings about it, and on the after-effects (physical, emotional, and spiritual) that I've been experiencing.

Following the recognized Standards Of Care,  I mailed to the surgeons of my choice (Drs. Yvon Menard and Pierre Brassard in Montreal) all the information their office had asked for:  a letter of recommendation from my psychologist stating her diagnosis and her assessment that surgery would be appropriate for me, a second opinion from a psychiatrist who also determined that surgery would be appropriate, copies of the psychological tests that had been done by a third specialist (Rorschach and MMPI tests), and a complete medical history.  This was in late June.

In early July I received a phone call from the office to say that my paperwork was in order and satisfactory and to set a surgery date.  I chose the middle of October because I thought it would take me that long to tie up all the loose ends that needed to be taken care of with work, family, friends, etc., and because October is a very auspicious month for me, a month in which several spiritual landmarks in my life have taken place.  I thought that it would also be appropriate as the month for my newest "rebirth".

During the three months that elapsed between scheduling surgery and my departure for Montreal, I made a very conscious effort *not* to put too much attention on it.  There were just too many things that needed to be done before surgery and I didn't want my energy and focus to be dissipated by anxieties, worries, eagerness, or euphoria about the approaching date.

Clients, a very long list of them whose jobs were in various stages of being completed, needed to be finished off so that I could spend my recuperation time recuperating rather than thinking about who might be impatiently drumming their fingers and waiting for me to get back to them.  Regular clients had to be told that I wouldn't be available for several months.  Family and friends needed to be notified of what would be happening, when, where, for how long, and where I could be reached during my stay in Montreal and afterwards during my recovery.  Mail needed to be temporarily forwarded to the friend's house where I would be staying after surgery.  There were no fewer than seven transgender speaking/educational engagements that I had agreed to do for various people and organizations.  There was a long list of medical tests that needed to be done before surgery and of items that I needed to buy either for my stay in Montreal or for my recovery time afterwards.  Pre-surgical visits with my electrologist, my psychologist, and my endocrinologist had to be arranged and made.  And finally, there were about 12 hours of audio recordings of a legal conference that I had promised a friend I would transcribe for her before I left for surgery. All of it kept me very, very busy.

But all of it could not prevent the inevitable, emotional realization that what I had been longing for, struggling for, and moving towards for nearly forty years was finally about to occur, and when the realization hit me, it hit with a wallop that I really wasn't expecting.

It came in the form of a card from one of my sisters, nothing special really, a typical greeting card with a few words written on the inside wishing me a speedy recovery and assurances that her thoughts were with me through the surgery. But within that short little paragraph were some words which hit me like a ton of bricks. I wrote about it in my notes:

> "I receive a card from my sister, Mary. She is
> wishing me well on my surgery and she says,
> among other things, 'I will miss my oldest
> brother ... but I welcome my new sister.' She is
> the first family member to say the words 'I will
> miss my...brother', and the floodgates are finally
> opened and I cry uncontrollably. My God, I will
> miss him too. He has been with me for so long;
> he has done so much to hold me together; he is
> so familiar; he guided me through his world ...
> our world; his spiritual arms enfolded me always
> in his love, and now I have reached the doorway
> and I know he can't come with me. He hands
> me over lovingly, willingly, to my new life ... but
> he must stay behind. Dear God, why must this
> be the price?"

My pain was not over anything physical. There was no worry or concern over the loss of a penis which, in my mind, had never really been a part of me. Rather, I had not realized what the mask had come to mean to me, how much that facade that I had held up for people to see had become a part of me, how much I had used it to protect me from the emotional pain of rejection, how it kept the world from knowing my "terrible" secret: that I was not and could not be who they wanted me to be.

There is in the human psyche an innate understanding about the nature of personal growth and evolution.  Every spiritual tradition has it.  In Christianity it is most highly expressed in the concept of the death and rebirth of Christ, a symbolic expression of the change that we must all go through in order to mature spiritually.  Classical mythology has it in the story of the Phoenix, the bird which rises to a new life from its own ashes.  Eastern religions express it in the inseparable connection between death and birth and the view that *both* are needed for the maintenance of existence and evolution ... in order for the flower to blossom, the bud must die.

I have learned that transsexuals, whatever their spiritual affiliation may be, are keenly aware of the transformational connection between death and birth.  By the time they are actually ready to successfully take that step into a new gender and a new sex, most have developed a personal, spiritual maturity which solidly encompasses the idea that a part of them will be dying for the greater good and growth of the rest of themselves.  Obviously, it is not a literal, physical death.  I am still here, as are 99% of the personality traits and characteristics that made me a man and which now make me a woman; but something *is* dead, some spiritual immaturity that had been a part of me for a very long time, and that death has given rise to the beginnings of a new kind of life.  The words "death" and "birth" do not really convey the idea, the impact, or the importance of the change, but they are the best that we can do with our limited vocabulary.

Within a single day, my realization and acceptance that a "death" was imminent had transformed me enough to do something I had never done before in my life.  In my notes I wrote:

"It is 11:00 p.m. and I am phoning my sister,
Mary.  I ask if she has a few minutes to talk with
me because 'I need to cry', and I tell her of my
sense of loss and my voice breaks and the tears
begin again.  In 44 years of living I cannot recall
ever having told anyone that I needed to cry,
and I can recall only a handful of times when I
cried and someone was there to comfort me.
Most of my crying has been done alone, internally, on the shoulder of my brother, Jean.  I
have kept it hidden so no one would know about
us.  I talk, and I cry, and Mary listens quietly and
occasionally speaks soft words.  Nothing is resolved, really, but I don't need resolution ... I
need release.  That old shoulder isn't there
anymore, and new shoulders need to be found.
It's a start."

It was not that there was no one around as I was growing up who would have tried to comfort me when I needed it, for
there were many such people, and many of them had given me
much love and comfort when I needed it for various reasons.
But I had never told anyone about my transsexuality.  It was the
secret that I never felt I could share with anyone because I was
afraid that it would make me unacceptable.  Because I couldn't
share it, I couldn't ask for help with it and, as a result, my fears
and anxieties and worries and insecurities about it had remained
for a lifetime uncomforted.

Over the next few days I told a lot of people how I was
feeling, and I cried a lot.  I cried whenever I thought about it.  I
cried when I talked with my mom and dad. I cried when I talked
with various friends.  I cried when I talked with a transsexual
friend of mine who is a psychiatric nurse, and I cried when I

talked about it with my therapist.  The last two folks showed definite signs of relief and both said the same thing: "I was worried
about you, but I feel better now.  If you had gotten all the way
through this and all the way up to Montreal and had never shown
any sense of loss or any ambiguous feelings about this really
momentous change that is about to take place in your life, then I
would have been really worried about how you would have dealt
with it all afterwards."

On the 6th of October I met with my therapist for the last
time before my surgery.  We talked about the sense of loss that I
was feeling and she helped me to understand how it fit into the
pattern of my life.  She suggested that I honor my past by taking
something with me to Montreal, some one item that I felt repre-
sented the old me and that would serve as a bridge between the
old and new eras of my life, thus reassuring me that what I
feared would be lost would actually always be available if I would
only ask for it.  It was a very good suggestion, and it took me
only a few moments to settle on the item it would be:  my Tran-
scendental Meditation ID badge, the little photo ID that is used to
get into the large group-meditation buildings during national con-
ferences.  The photo on it is twenty years old, definitely me in
"guy" mode, but the meditation that I was doing then is the same
meditation that I am doing today ... it has been with me through
everything and held me together for decades ... and I could not
think of a better reminder that change and stability always go
hand in hand.

I like my therapist.  She's a good therapist; she knows
the transgender subject matter; she's had a number of transgender clients over the years; I trust that she will not let any SRS
candidate just slide on through to surgery without being *very*
prepared, and as a result I have referred a number of trans folks
to her.  At that meeting I finally felt I could ask her the question
that I had been waiting to ask her for almost a year: "Am I the
first transgender client you've had who has made it as far as

surgery?"  When I asked, she got a big smile on her face and said, "*Yes*, and I feel very good about you.  You are ready.  You are as prepared as anyone could be for this, and I have no doubt that everything is going to go very well and that you are going to handle it wonderfully."  Then she gave me a little present, something representative of earth and growth and potential and femininity.  What that item was is not as important as the emotional and spiritual meaning that it had for me or as important as the gratitude I felt for the help she had been to me over the preceding three years, and I made sure that little present was among the very few extraneous things that I packed to take with me to Montreal.

The next day was spent running around and buying things that needed to be gotten for the two weeks in Montreal: medical supplies, clothing to wear during recuperation that I could bleed on and then wouldn't feel bad about throwing away, a small portable radio, getting American money changed to Canadian.  I also made last-minute phone calls and closed up the house (since I would be going to a friend's house after surgery and would not actually be home for nearly two months).  Late that afternoon and into the evening I did packing, finally getting everything I thought I would really need for a two-month absence into one large suitcase, a smallish duffle bag, and a small backpack kind of bag.  I finally got to bed at about 11:00 p.m. and actually managed to sleep quite soundly.

# COUNTDOWN TO SURGERY

**Five Days Before Surgery:**

My eyes opened, as they usually do, about 5:30 a.m. and I got up and began the final preparations for the day and the trip up to Montreal. I had made arrangements for a transgender friend of mine (whose femme name is Lucy) to drive me up in her car and she showed up at my house promptly at 8:00 a.m. only to find me behind schedule, and the two of us did not actually leave until about 8:45 a.m. As part of the "great plan", I had arranged for Lucy to stay at the residence with me for a night so that she wouldn't have to think about driving the seven hours back or paying for an expensive hotel room in Montreal. She expanded on the plan, however, and decided to spend a few days in Montreal "en femme" as a kind of mini-vacation. That was fine with me, as I knew that I would have a few days before entering the hospital and thought it would be fun to do a little sight-seeing with someone I knew.

In deference to my concerns about getting over the border as easily as possible, Lucy made our entrance into Canada in "guy mode" and at one of the more heavily traveled customs offices, where I expected that the idea of a transsexual entering the country would not throw them into a tizzy.

Five months earlier I had driven a friend of mine up to Montreal for the same surgery that I was now going up to have. At that time, when we reached the border, the questioning directed at her had gone something like this:

Q: Good morning.  Where are you going?
A: To Montreal.
Q: How long will you be staying?
A: For a couple of weeks.
Q: Are you going for business or pleasure?
A: A little of both.
Q: What is your business in Montreal?
A: I'm going up to have some surgery.
Q: Who will be paying for it?
A: I am.  It's all been paid for already.
Q: Do you have any kind of letter or documentation to that effect?
A: Yes I do.
Q: Very good.  Please pull up and park at the front of the building, go inside, and talk with the man at the counter.

My friend did as she was asked and the man at the counter looked at the letter provide by the surgeon stating that all the costs for surgery had been taken care of and the socialized medical establishment in Canada would not be paying anything. He then called out two other customs officers who also looked at the letter and asked my friend a few question about what kind of surgery she was having.  She was then asked to sit and wait while the three of them went into an office off to the side.  Some snickering was heard, and it seems that they called the clinic to verify that she was actually scheduled for surgery and that it was paid for.  After that, they returned her letter and let her go.  The whole process took about 20 minutes, and I was expecting the same thing to happen with me.

Instead, what happened was that we pulled up to the customs office, with my friend driving, and the conversation went something like this:

> Q: Good morning.  Where are you going?
> A: To Montreal.
> Q: How long will you be staying?
> A: Just a few days.  (I leaned forward to let the customs agent know that I would be staying for a few weeks, but she ignored me.)
> Q: Are you going for business or pleasure?
> A: Pleasure.  (I tried to interject that I was going to be having some surgery, but the agent ig-nored me.)
> Q: Are you bringing any alcohol or cigarettes into the country?
> A: No.
> Q: Thank you.  Enjoy your stay.  (And my friend drove us through.)

The whole process took less than a minute.  We were just a guy and his babe going up to the big city for some fun and nothing else needed to be known about us.  Part of me thought, "Well, that was easy!"  Another part of me thought, "Hey wait a minute!  Don't I matter in any of this!?"  It was obvious that, as a woman, I didn't, and I couldn't decide if I should be upset about it or not.  Was this a benefit for ease of international travel or an affront to my value as a person ... or was it both, an example of the very strange mish-mash of benefits and responsibilities that we assign to the different genders in our cultures and which most of us never really question and are never really aware of?

Ultimately, I decided that this particular issue wasn't important enough to get upset about.  I had wanted to get into Canada as easily as possible and had done so without any deception on my part, so I decided that any affront created by the customs agent's assumption was something that could be overlooked.  We all have to pick and choose our battles, and this just wasn't a battle that I needed or wanted to engage in.

Two hours later we were crossing the bridge going into Montreal and merging into the beginning of the rush-hour traffic.  It was about 4:00 p.m. when we finally arrived at the residence where I would be staying for several days before surgery and for about a week after leaving the hospital.  Let me set the scene for you, so that you can have a better idea of what the Montreal experience is like.

SRS in Montreal is actually accomplished in three different places.  Right in the middle of town is the business office.  From here all of the telephoned, written, and emailed requests for information are answered, brochures and forms are sent out, payments are collected, scheduling is done, data files and patient records are kept and updated, the doctors have their offices, and a small amount of minor outpatient surgery is done.  Actually, I've never even seen this building, though I've called and written to the staff there a number of times.

About five miles away is the actual clinic/hospital where surgery is done.  It is a squat, square, white, two-story building with its basement buried only half way in the ground so that natural light can get to that floor as well.  One goes up the front steps into the lobby area and straight ahead to the receptionist's desk, behind which is the nurse's station.  Patient rooms line the perimeter of the first floor with the nurse's station right in the middle of everything.  In the front, right-hand corner of the building are two rooms and one bathroom which comprise the transgender

"wing" of the clinic.  Drs. Menard and Brassard have made
transsexual surgery a kind of specialty within their practice, but
they also do a complete line of plastic and reconstructive surgery
for non-transgendered clients as well, which is why only two of
the ten or twelve patient rooms are set aside for SRS.  Each patient room has two hospital-style beds, two small dressers with
their tops just about level with the top of the bed, a small closet,
a TV, and a curtain that can be drawn between the beds.  The
operating rooms are located on the second floor.  Somewhere in
the building is the laundry and kitchen.  About the only things I
ever saw in this building were the two bedrooms, the bathroom,
the nurse's station, the hallway which was a buffer between the
nurse's station and the patient rooms, the prep room where patients lie on gurneys waiting to be wheeled into the operating
room, and the ceiling of the operating room.

The third and most important building of the three is the
residence.  When I had surgery, the residence was located on
the north side of the island of Montreal proper, just a ten minute
walk from the clinic.  To its east were private, suburban houses,
closely packed together.  Directly behind it was a small cul-de-
sac surrounded by more cute little suburban houses.  Beyond
those houses was the river.  To the west of the residence was a
huge, modern, six-story apartment building, and to the west of
that a big hospital and then a park which borders the river and
contains a paved walking path along the shore.

Directly across the street from the residence, beginning
about a block before the residence building and going past the
apartment building, the hospital, and the park was the provincial
prison which looked mostly like a huge, green space surrounded
by a chain-link fence with an island of gray and brown stone in
the middle of it.  This was a minimum security prison, and the
staff at the residence told us that on the weekends you can
sometimes see some of the inmates (with their brown-bag
lunches) walking out of the prison on weekend leave.

The residence itself was a low, split-level-style building with a stone and natural wood veneer, an attached two-car garage, and a six-foot high wooden fence enclosing the backyard area.  In one section of the building were two levels containing a total of five client bedrooms, the doctor's office, and the big, main bathroom.  In the basement area was the laundry, a smaller bathroom, and the sleeping quarters for whichever staff member was on duty that night.  The remainder of the building was made up of a *huge*  living room and the kitchen and dining area.  The entire north wall of the living room was floor-to-ceiling glass, interrupted in the middle by a very large stone fireplace.  A sliding glass door on the east wall led to the roofed patio and from there to the backyard with its in-ground, cement swimming pool (which took up half of the fenced-in area).

The south wall of the large, modern kitchen was all glass from about three feet above the floor up to the ceiling, and a skylight was located above the dining area table, making the whole room sunny and warm.  A door from the dining area went to the attached garage, which doubled as the smoking area in inclement weather when the patio became unusable.

Going up the stairs to the second-level area, one came immediately upon the doorway to the large bathroom which contained a toilet with an attached bidet, an enclosed shower with multiple shower heads, a two-sink vanity over which was a very-well-lighted six-foot-long mirror, and a raised jacuzzi tub.  Over the tub was a skylight which made the room bright and sunny.  In the hallway to the left of the bathroom door was a black, ebony dresser with colorful, painted and inlaid birds and flowers on it.

Turning right at the top of the stairs, one entered the second-level hallway, actually a walkway, which was open on one side to the living-room space below and which, on the other side, led into each of the three bedrooms on the second level. The front and middle bedrooms each had two beds with night stands and a small closet.  The back bedroom, which was about twice as large, had three beds with night stands, two closets, a big picture window to the back yard, and a doorway which opened onto a small balcony.

I was familiar with the place because, as I have said, I drove a friend of mine there only five months earlier and got to spend the night before returning home.  I was also familiar with the house rules (which a staff person usually tells to each new arrival while there are giving the tour of the place):

***  You must be back in the building by 10:00 p.m. each night.

***  If you leave the premises you are expected to tell a staff person where you are going and when you expect to be back.

***  If you will not be present for one of the meals, you are expected to let the chef know ahead of time.

***  Laundry is done for you once a day.  Dirty clothes must be left in the basket in the basement laundry by 12:00 noon to get done that day.  Bloodied undergarments should be placed in the special bucket provided (containing water and bleach) so that they can be completely cleaned and disinfected.  Clean clothes are put on the second-level dresser outside the bathroom, where you may pick them up.

***  No smoking is allowed anywhere inside the building.  You may smoke on the patio by the pool or, in bad weather, in the garage area where a table and chairs are set up.

***  You may watch TV or videos if you wish, but are expected to keep the volume sufficiently low after 10:00 p.m. so that folks who want to may sleep.

***  Meals are served at 8:00 a.m., 12:00 noon, and 6:00 p.m.

*** The kitchen is off-limits to grazers after 10:00 p.m.

*** Telephone calls can be received, and outgoing credit-card calls can be made, on the cordless living-room phone dedicated for the clients.  Incoming and outgoing calls should be limited to 15 minutes so that others can use the phone as well.

*** Do *not* lock the bathroom door while you are in there.  This is so staff people can reach help post-operative clients if the client has problems while in the bathroom.

*** To prevent possible post-operative infection, both sides of the toilet seat must be cleaned and disinfected after every use.

*** Never go out onto the street except in street clothes (i.e. do not parade in front of the public wearing your pajamas).

*** Post-operative clients are given preference in bathroom and comfortable-furniture use.

When Lucy and I finally got to the residence we were warmly greeted and shown to our room.  One of the staff people gave Lucy the tour, and the rules, while I got settled in.  Usually, I would have been assigned as my roommate whoever was going to have SRS on the same day that I did.  However, because I had Lucy staying with me for one night, and because my roommate-to-be had made plans to have one of her sisters with her for several days leading up to and through surgery, I essentially had a private room for the four days before I went to the clinic.

Still, it was only twenty minutes or so before I got to meet my future surgical and post-operative roommate.  Her name is Anne-Marie (she told me to call her Anne), she is about three years older than me, the same height and weight, and has hair that is the same dark-brown color as mine but shorter.  She seemed a little quiet and reserved in her new surroundings, as I am sure I must have seemed as well, but I could tell from her easy smile and the twinkle in her eyes that underneath she was both excited and had a lively personality.

We introduced ourselves to each other and began the strange little ritual that most transgender people go through when they first meet each other in surroundings where they can speak freely without fear of any kind of social recrimination: we started telling each other about our transgender lives and what is has been like growing up transgender.  One of the things that makes this little, usually unrecognized, ritual so strange is the fact that we always know exactly what the other person is going to say.  We know it because most of us, regardless of our present or past circumstances, have all had pretty much the same experiences of confusion, fear, guilt, anxiety, struggle, etc.  Most of us began to experience our transgenderism at about the same time in life and most of us struggled with it in the same, limited variety of ways.  Most of us have the same feelings about it and about ourselves as transgender people, and most of us worked through very similar confusions in the same, fairly predictable, series of self-revelations.  Those of us who have gone as far as surgery have done so because of the same feelings and desires. In many (but by no means all) respects, we are multiple copies of the same book.

The second thing that makes this little ritual so strange is the fact that the information isn't being exchanged to inform, but rather to validate.  It's kind of like in those old black-and-white, World War II, prisoner-of-war movies where the leader of the prisoners is grilling a new inmate to make sure he is not a planted spy: "Who won the pennant in 1934?"  Only a real American would know that, right?  With transgender folks, I think the exchange of life experiences serves to validate who we are to others like us and let them know that we can be open and trusting of each other.  Anyway, it seems to have worked with us because we bonded almost instantly.

I am sure the fact that we also shared other personality traits, preferences, life experiences, and world-views was a big help as well.  Within minutes we had synchronized our understanding of what much of our two-week stay would hold in store for us and what we hoped to get out of it beyond the simple change in anatomy.  It is so much easier to get along with someone when the two of you are on the same "wavelength", and I knew then that whatever the next two weeks would bring, we could count on each other for any needed physical, emotional, or spiritual support.

Anne and I (both male-to-female) were the only two people scheduled for surgery that week.  The three folks who were there the week before us consisted of Phillippa and Claudia (both male-to-female), and Lee (a female-to-male whose wife, Barbara, was with him for his three week stay).

The way the schedule is set up at the residence is such that much of the time you will have both pre-operative and post-operative folks staying there.  Anne and I were the only two pre-ops who would arrive that day (Thursday) for surgery the following Tuesday.  The next day (Friday) the post-ops from the clinic would return to the residence.  The two groups (pre and post) would then get to interact with and help each other for about three days before Anne and I moved over to the clinic.  Two days after our surgery, the previous group of post-ops would leave for home and a new group of pre-ops would arrive.  The day after they arrived, Anne and I would return to the residence and the whole cycle would repeat itself.  Inserted into this ongoing cycle are occasional folks who arrive and only spend a few days at the residence while having some other, less intrusive, surgery performed (e.g. breast augmentation, beard removal, voice surgery, etc.)  All in all, it is really a wonderfully orchestrated schedule that allows folks to both know and help each other, physically and emotionally.  Pre-ops are always asking questions of the post-ops, and post-ops are always offering their stories and thoughts on a variety of things from diet to comfortable sleeping positions.

Anne, Lucy, and I spent the next hour and half settling into our rooms and talking with each other.  At dinner time we all gathered at the dining table, together with the staff members who were on duty at the time.  Dr. Menard and his wife, Sylvia, came over from the clinic and joined us as well.  It was very much like an old-fashioned family dinner, with everyone talking about a variety of subjects and getting to know each other better.  Almost immediately, mealtime became a kind of healing ritual with our little family of post-ops, pre-ops, staff, doctors, family members, and friends...whoever was at the house when it was time to eat ... all sitting together and sharing their thoughts and experiences.  Sometimes the talk was about surgery or recuperation or transgender life experiences, sometimes it was about politics, fishing trips, cosmopolitan life-styles, art, jobs, or whatever else would pop up for discussion.  All of it helped to lift our spirits and give us support not only because we knew that the other people around us were familiar with our experience and accepting of each of us as individuals, but also because the warm, laid-back, home-like surroundings were much more conducive to healing (on a psychological level) than a cold and sterile hospital room or hotel room would have been.

After dinner, three or four of us sat around talking for a while.  It had been another long day for me, and I wanted to get as much rest as I could in the few remaining days before surgery, so I decided to call it quits at about 9:00 p.m. and went upstairs to bed.

**Four Days Before Surgery:**

Besides trying to rest and relax before surgery, the two or three days after someone first arrives at the residence are also spent being tourists and seeing the sights of Montreal, a kind of psychological diversion and mini-vacation.  Because there are not too many exciting things to do at the residence besides eat, sleep, read, watch TV, and sit on the patio; and because everyone realizes that they are not going to be able to do anything other than that after surgery, it is usually not very difficult to get the pre-op folks to take advantage of the time to paint the town red ... or at least a light shade of pink.  Several of the staff had regaled us with stories of some of the previous pre-op patients who had stayed out on the town all night, hitting all the bars and dance clubs.  Since I'm not much of a dancer and don't care for bars I was satisfied with something a little more sedate, and I was happy to find both Anne and Lucy equally interested in more laid-back activities.  After breakfast we decided to break ourselves in slowly with a walk to a nearby shopping center to pick up some supplies and do a little window shopping.  "Nearby" turned out to be about a mile away, but it was a sunny and warm fall morning, so the three hours we spent on our little excursion were really quite fun.

We got back just in time for lunch.  Joining us for the noontime meal was Barbara, the wife of the FTM person who had his surgery during the previous week.  He was still in the clinic, as were the two MTF folks, but Barbara was staying at the residence while he was in the hospital and she joined us for meals along with everyone else.  The reason I hadn't seen her before was because she had come back from the clinic after I had gone to bed the previous night and had left to go back to the clinic before I was downstairs that morning.  Anyway, she was just a dear person, bright and cheerful, with a wonderful southern drawl and a nice sense of humor.  Over lunch we talked a bit about their experience and how Lee, her husband, was doing, then she was off for the clinic again.  Anne, Lucy, and I were left to our own devices.

We told Raphael (the chef at the residence) that we would be back in time for dinner and then headed out to see the famous "underground city" of Montreal, a collection of underground malls and shopping areas in various points around the downtown that allow the Montrealians (or is it Montrealers?) to go about their usual business in the dark of winter without having to spend a lot of time out in the cold.  Lucy had been to the city several times before, so she directed our travels on the subway system, around town, and into the subterranean meccas.  I'll be honest with you; I'm not a good mall rat, and several hours of malling in crowded places with little or no natural light was more than enough to satisfy me.  One of the things I had specifically planned to *not* do in Montreal was spend a lot of money, so even if there had been a lot of stuff that I liked (and there wasn't), I would not have bought anything ... especially anything that I would have had to turn around and carry home with me.  Still, it was interesting to see the subway system (*very* clean and very organized), the range of architecture around the city (colonial stonework to modern glass cubes), the variety of stores (clothing stores, especially, leaned heavily towards European styling), and the number of eateries (the folks in Montreal obviously *love* culinary variety).  We got back to the residence at about 4:00 p.m.

I had made arrangements for Lucy to stay at the residence with me for one night in exchange for driving me to the city, expecting that she would want to leave to return home the next morning.  But, since she was in the mood to make it a weekend in the big city, and since I couldn't afford to pay for her to stay more nights with me, she decided to go in search of a little Bed & Breakfast somewhere.  At dinner the previous evening she had asked about various places, and almost as soon as we got back to the residence she and I were back out on the road, this time in her car, to look at the place that had been most highly recommended.  It turned out to be a wonderful little house across the river from the residence, with a park right across the street, a spacious sunroom on the second floor, and an enclosed back yard with a little pond, a flower garden, and a deck for dining when the weather was warmer.  Lucy's room was nearly a suite, with a huge bed area, an equally huge sitting area, and a private bath.  She couldn't have found a nicer place.  We got her settled and then returned to the residence by about 5:00 p.m.

Shortly after our return, the new post-ops came back from the clinic.  I was sitting in the living room, around the corner from the entryway, and so did not see Barbara and Lee as they came in and went right to their first-level room.  Claudia and Phillippa, however, were in the back bedroom on the second level and had to come within view as they made their way up the stairs.  Both of them had the strangest combination of looks on their faces: sparkling eyes and huge grins (like cats who just got a canary) coupled with gritted teeth and frequent flinches as they moved slowly towards their destination.  They were also joking with each other, their conversation spotted with little groans of pain and such admonitions as "Please ... don't make me laugh!" or "I'll get you for that."  I'd never seen two people who were obviously in so much pain being so happy about it.  The two of them stopped by the living room long enough for all of us to introduce ourselves and for them to assure us that "it" was really a "wonderful experience", and then they excused themselves to go rest a bit and disappeared into their room, joking and groaning the whole way.  I seem to recall that Anne and I just kind of looked at each other.

Dinner that evening had a decidedly different tenor to it from our previous meals.  Lee was able to join us all, though he was obviously in a good deal of pain (not too surprising when you realize that FTM surgery takes two doctors 7 1/2 hours to complete while MTF surgery takes one doctor 2 1/2 hours to do).

He came in, walking very slowly, and leaning on Barbara for support.  According to the house rules, the post-ops were given preference as to which seats they wanted at the table.  Lee and Phillippa took the two end seats because those had a little more room around them and so where easier to get into and out of, while Claudia (who seemed to be doing better as far as pain and motion was concerned) took a side seat close to the end of the table.  Barbara sat across from her, right next to Lee, so that she could help him if he needed it.  Pre-ops, guests, and staff took the remaining seats.

Watching the post-ops move into place and sit down was enough to give one pause as to what the future was going to hold.  They moved very slowly and deliberately, taking small steps.  Pillows, and inflatable rubber "donuts" were in everyone's arms when they arrived, and everyone seemed to have their own combination and order for placing the cushions on the chairs before sitting down.  When they sat, they slowly lowered themselves onto the seat, often making two or three attempts before finally finding a position that was bearable and usually biting their lips or clenching their teeth during the whole process.  If someone was having a particularly painful day he or she might not even try to sit, opting instead to stand at the counter or lean against the wall with the plate in one hand and a fork in the other.  None of that should have been very surprising to us because not only were the three post-ops dealing with a variety of stitches and skin grafts in some rather tender places, but Claudia and Phillippa still had surgical stents sewn into them to help keep the new vaginas open, Lee had several drainage tubes coming out of his groin area, and all three of them still had catheters inserted.

None of the post-ops ate much food, especially Phillippa who had made the mistake of eating quite a bit while in the clinic and whose stomach juices turned out to be slow at making a comeback.  The result was that she was quite bound up with a stomach full of food that didn't seem to be going anywhere.  Lee was still quite weak and in pain from his experience and didn't have the use of his left arm because of the skin grafting that had been done there.  Nevertheless, all three of them ate something, and in the days to follow we could see their appetites improving each day.

The dinner talk that night was mostly about the surgical experience and the two or three days afterwards, and the post-ops all seemed to be particularly eager to tell their stories and share whatever helpful information they could pass along to us.  Questions, thoughts, and suggestions flew hot and heavy for the next 30 or 40 minutes until the three of them had their fill of food and talk and, one by one, excused themselves to find more comfortable positions and to rest.

An hour or so later Marie-Andree, one of the staff people, pulled out a video and asked us if we wanted to see it.  Because I knew three other transsexuals who had been through Montreal for their surgeries, I knew exactly what it was.  It was a video of the male-to-female surgical process in all it's medical gory .... sorry, I mean glory.  Every major incision, retraction, suture, and graft of the process was shown in close-up detail with a narration by Dr. Menard of what he was doing with each move.  A similar video of the female-to-male procedure also exists, but since Anne and I were both MTF, that is the one that they offered to show us.  Both Anne and I *did* want to see it, so it was popped into the machine in the living room and the two of us and Lucy sat and watched.  I remember Anne reclining on one of the couches with her right hand over her mouth, occasionally biting her index finger, while I sat quietly watching.  Lucy would interject something light-hearted every now and then to break the palpable tension, and at times one of us would ask the others about something that wasn't quite clear or we would throw in remarks like, "Oh, so that's how he does that!  I always wondered."

The tales from the clinic that the post-ops shared with us, the video we were now watching, and the interaction with the post-ops over several days were a sobering combination, and that is exactly what they were supposed to be.  These last few days before surgery were more than just a chance to rest.  They were also designed to be an opportunity for the pre-ops to learn what the surgical process and its aftermath were really like and to reflect on what they were about to do.  The surgeons wanted to do their best to make sure that no one went into SRS with misperceptions about what the medical process was going to be like.  This is not to say that no one has ever gone into SRS with misperceptions about what the *psychological* process would be like, but that is not the surgeon's concern ... that is something that the mandated psychological therapy before surgery is supposed to have prepared the individual for.  Clearly, however, from a medical standpoint, the doctors try to make sure that their clients are as prepared as they can be for the rigors of their surgery and that they have the best opportunity to begin healing afterwards.

**Three Days Before Surgery:**

The next day, Saturday, was another tourist day for the pre-ops.  Lucy came over from her B&B after breakfast and, after we let Raphael know that Anne and I would not be there for lunch, the three of us piled into the car and drove into the city to take in the Montreal Botanical Gardens and the Museum of Fine Art.

It was actually a very low-key day for all of us.  The weather was foggy and rainy, so we were restricted to walking through the seven huge greenhouses at the gardens rather than enjoying any of the outdoor acreage that would otherwise have been available.  I particularly enjoyed the Japanese greenhouse with its formal garden in the center and the dozens of bonsai plants around its perimeter, a few of them more than 100 years old.

After that we drove to the Museum of Fine Art, parked the car, and went in search of someplace to have lunch before continuing.  What we found was a cozy little bistro, one of those hole-in-the-wall places with lots of ambiance and reasonable prices, where we were able to get some really good soup (I had hot borscht, sweet and sour and delicately seasoned, with a dollop of sour cream on top) and a couple of pizzas.  We took our time, discussing a variety of things including our impending surgery, and then ambled the remaining couple of blocks to the museum where we had a pleasant, but uneventful, afternoon.

We returned to the residence in time for supper and more pleasant discussion and then, that evening, watched a video of a show that had appeared on the ARTS & ENTERTAINMENT channel a few days before, a show about the transgender community.  We all agreed that it was one of the most balanced presentations that we had ever seen done by a major producer.

**Two Days Before Surgery:**

The next morning, Sunday, Lucy came by the residence long enough to say good-bye and then headed back to Maine.  I had already begun to feel more need to center myself, relax, and become more contemplative, and her departure was in some ways welcomed as I really didn't feel that I wanted to be touristing for yet another day.  Anne, too, was feeling more reclusive and in need of more rest and, since her sister was due to arrive that evening, she and I agreed that we would spend the day being really laid-back.  The most exciting thing we did that day was to make the one-mile trek to the shopping center to buy some toothpaste for me and a few other items that Claudia needed.  We walked and talked and compared our feelings about the ordeal that we were soon to go through.  Both of us were uncertain and anxious about the pain that we would obviously be experiencing.  Yet, at the same time, we knew that we really had no other alternative because we had already, in our lives, tried everything else we could think of to become the people that we were intended to be, and we knew that only the actual, physical transformation would ultimately bring that about.  There was no euphoria, and no illusion that our lives would be perfect afterwards, only the determination to proceed that comes from the conviction that a certain, skewed piece of our lives had to be brought into alignment in order for us to be more balanced and more whole.

We spent the day resting and talking.  I read a bit and took a nap.  When Phillippa and Claudia were around we picked their brains for a more in-depth description about what they had experienced and were now going through and how they handled it.  Of course, there was no guarantee that we would experience all the same things that they did, or be able to handle them in the same way, but knowing what was possible was psychologically fortifying and I was glad that they were around.

Phillippa's intestinal blockage (and the three days of great discomfort she had from it) had ended the evening before when she finally had a sizable bowel movement ... something that both she and the staff had been anxiously awaiting.  She had definitely become more lively afterwards, but now both she and Claudia seemed to be fighting with the next adversary, the pain and discomfort created by the fact that their bodies were beginning to regain more sensation in the groin area and were not at all happy to have urinary catheters hanging out of them and vaginal stents sewn into them.  They both were moving even more slowly, grimacing more frequently, taking pain pills as often as the staff would allow, and had a definite preference for lying down or standing rather than sitting.  Through a forced smile Phillippa said, "Oh, it's not that bad.  It just feels like someone parked a tractor-trailer in there."  Relief was on the way, however, as they were both scheduled to have the catheters and stents removed early the next morning.

Phillippa's experience with having a lot of food in her stomach throughout her stay in the clinic only gave me added incentive to put a plan of my own into action.  I had already asked Dr. Menard if he had any objections to me fasting before going in for surgery.  He said he didn't have a problem with it because he didn't think it would matter one way or the other.  I, however, *did* think it would matter and had already resolved to go onto a liquid diet two days before my surgery was scheduled.  I did not want my body spending a lot of energy digesting food when it needed to be spending it on healing, and I certainly did not want the situation that Phillippa had.  Sylvia, who was a nurse, expressed doubt that it was a good thing to do because she felt that the patients should have a good, steady diet (especially of protein) to help them recuperate.  And Raphael, the chef, who had looked askance at the fact that I was vegetarian, had an even harder time believing that I was actually *not* going to eat.  But I had already bought the supplies two days before ... a variety of fruit and vegetable juices, flavored protein mixes to put into milk, and veggie bullion cubes ... so they saw that I was serious about the idea and simply shrugged their shoulders and, I'm sure, wondered what the crazy vegetarian person might try next.  Anne and my surgeries were scheduled for Tuesday morning, so I started my liquid fast on Sunday morning.  At first everyone was asking me, "Gosh, is that *all* you're going to eat?", but once I explained my reasoning to them they all seemed to think it was a good idea, especially Phillippa, and by dinner time no one was batting an eye as I sat there with my glass of whatever and helped them pass the food around.

Anne's sister, Cindy, was due to arrive from Florida just after dinner, so Anne had joined us to eat quickly and then gone off to the airport to meet Cindy when she got in.  I grabbed my book, secluded myself in my room, and sat reading until they returned, which was about 8:00 p.m. because the plane had been delayed somewhere or other.  Cindy's decision to be in Montreal while Anne was having SRS was doubly meaningful to my roommate not only because it showed how much she was cared for and accepted, but also because the two of them had not actually seen each other in five years, since before Anne had begun her transition.  Such family acceptance is, unfortunately, not at all common within the transgender community, but when they finally got back it did not take me long to realize that Cindy was herself not at all common.  Standing perhaps half a head shorter than me, she had shoulder-length dark-blond hair, a fine tan, inquiring eyes that seemed always to want to know something new, an impish smile, and a life-is-cool aura that made her a pleasure to be around.  She had managed to get away from her husband and her job to join Anne for about five days, and it was obvious that the five years they had been apart had not dampened how much they cared about each other.

Cindy was introduced around and we all sat visiting and talking for a while until I began to feel tired.  I had just excused myself and gone to my room when Marie-Andree called to me from down by the office; it was time to sign releases.  This part I was aware of as well from my friend who had had her surgery six months earlier.  We went into the office, closed the door, and sat at the desk.  Marie-Andree passed me the releases, four or five pages of them, and I began to read.  As I recall, there was a statement on my part acknowledging that I had correctly followed the requirements for psychological therapy, hormone treatment, and full-time living that are part of the established Standards of Care.  There was a moderate amount of detail about what the surgery would entail: castration, removal of the penis, surgical formation of a vagina, loss of any ability to have children, and a statement saying that I had read and understood those facts.  And finally, there was a statement that the surgeon could not guarantee either a complete return of sensation or ability to have orgasm or that there would be no complications from surgery, and a statement that I understood those things.  I carefully read through all of it and signed in the required places.  Then I was asked for the $50 that we had been told would be needed for our pain medications after surgery, the ones we would be taking when we returned to the residence and which we would take with us when we went home.  Marie-Andree then asked me if I had any money or valuables that I wanted to store in the safe while I was in the clinic.  After that, I returned to my room and went to bed, my mind somewhat anxious about how much pain I might be in after surgery.

**One Day Before Surgery:**

The next morning, Monday, the day before surgery, Dr. Menard arrived about 7:00 a.m. and removed Claudia's and Phillippa's catheters and stents, and Sylvia had then instructed them in how to dilate and douche (I will be talking about that process a little later), so by the time Claudia and Phillippa showed up at the breakfast table they were all smiles and cheery, clearly in much less pain than the previous evening, and thrilled about being able to begin experiencing their new vaginas.  Much of the table talk that morning was about the relief from pain, dilating, douching, vaginas, and clitorises, and Barbara and Sylvia and Cindy (who had been born with their female anatomies) were making sure to put in their thoughts and observations as well.  Lee just shook his head and, in his sweet southern drawl, said, "I'll tell ya, I'm learnin' more about female anatomy than I *ever* wanted to know!"

Anne and I were both rather subdued and reflective that day, and Claudia, Phillippa, and Lee were very supportive and reassuring that everything would go well.  It was another day of low-key activity, quiet talks, contemplation, and naps for me.  In the afternoon Anne and I and Cindy went for a long walk through the park and along the river, and I seem to recall that, among other things, there was a lot of talk and consideration about our lives up until then and all the things that had led us to where we were now.

We got back from our walk about an hour or so before dinner and began to prepare for going into the clinic.  We'd been given a list of things that we would need while there (Claudia and Phillippa and Lee had given us their thoughts on what we would *actually* use and what we could leave behind), and those things needed to be put in the small overnight bag we would take with us.  The rest of our belongings had to be packed away and put in the office for safe-keeping because we would be together in a different room when we got back, while the rooms we were presently in would be given to the pre-ops who would arrive on Thursday.  We had to give ourselves enemas (the first of two), and we had to shave off all of our pubic hair....everything from the anus to almost the belly-button.  I knew about the shaving requirement ahead of time and had done it before even leaving for Montreal, which made it much easier to go back over it again that afternoon.  Of course, there were some areas that were a little difficult to see and reach with a razor, so Anne and I had agreed that when we were done we would check each other out and take care of anything that had been missed.  We are both fairly private people, and despite the reason for doing it, we both still found that having someone else handling our penises and scrotums and then coming at them with a razor was somewhat disquieting.  The experience did, however, help a little to prepare us psychologically for the remainder of our stay by bringing home a point that Claudia and Phillippa and all my other post-op friends had mentioned:  Once you go in for surgery, forget about holding on to any modesty.  In the hospital, all kinds of people are going to need to be touching you and doing all kinds of things to you, and back at the residence the staff will need to be asking you all kinds of questions, keeping an eye on you, and even checking your bathroom habits and dilating procedure.  It's all necessary, and you're just going to have to put up with it.

Dinner was pleasant and upbeat, with folks telling humorous stories about their lives and themselves and Cindy showing us photos of her and her husband swimming with a dolphin somewhere in Florida.  I sat with my glass of vegetable juice and Anne (who had decided that she liked the idea of eating less before surgery) eating a variety of fruit.

When we were done (about 7:00 p.m.), we went to our rooms, got our hospital bags, hauled our suitcases and other luggage into the office, put on our coats, hugged everyone amid lots of well-wishing, and then walked out the door and headed for the clinic with Cindy joining us.  When we arrived, we walked up the front steps and, finding the door locked, rang the bell.  I had a quick vision in my mind of Dorothy, the scarecrow, the tin-man, and the lion ringing the bell to the gates of the Emerald City, wanting to get in to see the wizard.  Through the glass door we could see a nurse appear at the receptionist's desk and a second later the buzz of the electric lock ushered us into the building.

The place was very quiet ... hey, what would you expect in a hospital at 8:00 p.m ... and the nurse at the desk was very pleasant.  We handed her our admissions papers (which had been given to us just before we left the residence) and said, "I think you're expecting us."  She replied, "Oh yes, we're expecting you."

She grabbed a clip-board and showed us to the room we would be in.  We waited expectantly as she checked the clip-board and announced, "Anne-Marie, you have the bed over by the window."  Then she smiled and said, "I suppose you know what that means?"  Oh yes, we knew what that meant because every post-op we'd talked to had let us in on the little secret.  For some reason, the arrangement in the clinic is that the person whose bed is by the window is the first person to go into surgery in the morning.  Don't ask me *how* they make the determination that one person should go before another or what factors they consider before deciding that, but the decision is made for us, it's not something that we get to decide between ourselves.  Anyway, that meant that I would have to hang out in the room (being anxious, worried, eager, bored, whatever) for a good part of the morning while Anne slept through her surgery.  "Take a few minutes to settle in," the nurse said, "and when you're ready, please come out to the nurse's station, one at a time, to fill out admissions forms."  Then she left.

Anne and I looked around.  It was just a typical hospital room ... I mean, what else were we expecting ... so we started to unpack our things and find places for them.  As we worked, Anne and Cindy and I were talking about the building and the room and asking each other about the placement of various things. We knew that for at least a couple of days we would not be out of the beds and that anything we would really want should be within arm's reach.  We also knew that once we were allowed out of the beds we would *not* be allowed to do any bending over, so things ought not to go into lower dresser drawers.  And, we knew that we would probably be quite weak and so should not have to do a lot of moving to get to various things.  I couldn't move my dresser closer to the bed, so I wheeled the bed closer to the dresser, allowing me to reach the dresser top from the bed. Onto the dresser top (nearest the bed) went tissues, my little radio with headphones, a glass of water, and the little change purse that held my ID's and my phone calling card.  On the other end of the dresser top went soap, shampoo, toothpaste, toothbrush, etc.  Clothes that I would need to reach when it came time to leave the clinic went into the top drawer where I could get at them without bending over too much.  The wastebasket went in front of the dresser, right by the tissues, and my slippers went on the floor on the other side of the bed where I could step into them almost as I stepped out of bed.  My bathrobe was thrown over the nearby chair, where it could be grabbed as I walked out of the room.  Anne wondered if the TV worked and I quickly replied that if she turned it on I would kill her.  She laughed and said that she really didn't want to watch it anyway.

I was ready, but Anne was ready before me.  Cindy gave me a hug and said that she would be back the next day, after surgery, to see how we were doing, and then Anne walked with her to the front door, stopping by the nurse's station after Cindy was gone.  I continued puttering with the placement of things and trying to find a decent station on the radio, waiting for Anne to get back.  When she finally returned I headed for my little interview.  The nurse went over all the information she had, double-checking all of it, especially the section on allergies and negative reactions to various medications.  She also asked for a contact name and phone number for "someone" related to me in case of some kind of emergency, and I gave her my father's.  Then she took my pulse and blood pressure, put one of those plastic name bracelets on me, handed me the second enema kit (letting me know that I should self-administer it before going to bed), gave me a sedative pill to help me sleep, asked me if I had any questions (I didn't), and that was then end of my admissions.

There really wasn't a whole lot left for Anne and me to say to each other at that point.  We engaged in small talk while getting undressed.  By then it was nearly 9:00 p.m.  Anne's surgery would start at 8:00 a.m. the next morning, mine sometime around 11:00, and since we both wanted to be rested we decided to go right to bed.  She went into the bathroom to do her enema and I went in to do mine as soon as she returned, then we both took our sleeping pills and got into bed.  The last thing we did was ask each other if we were ready, and upon hearing that we both *were*, we said good-night, turned over, and went to sleep.

# SURGERY AND THE HOSPITAL STAY

**Surgery Day:**

Surprisingly, we both actually slept.  I was awakened the next morning by the nurse saying, "Anne-Marie, it's time for you to get ready."  I watched as Anne was handed one of those surgical robes to put on (you know the ones, all front, no back) and as she proceeded to get herself undressed.  Then the anesthesiologist came in, gave her a shot in the thigh, and left, letting her know that he would be back in a few minutes.  Anne lay back on the bed and then turned her head towards me and said, "Well, I guess this is it."  I nodded and reassured her that everything would go fine.  Then, after a pause, I asked, "Can I have your Porsche if you don't come back?"  The shot she'd gotten was quickly taking effect and she was obviously starting to zone out.  Still, she chuckled and said, "Absolutely!"

At that point the anesthesiologist brought in a gurney and asked Anne to get onto it.  She climbed aboard, lay back, and was covered with a sheet up to her chest.  "I'll see you later," she said as he wheeled her out.  "I'm thinking of you," I answered as she disappeared out the door.

I thought I would spend the next two and a half hours being wide awake and anxious, but after wondering for a while what was going on in the operating room I fell back into sleep and didn't wake up until the nurse's voice came floating through the air saying, "Jean, it's your turn."  When I sat up in bed, she gave me the robe (all front, no back) and said that the anesthesiologist would be in to see me in a few minutes.  I asked her what time it was and was told "11:40".  I put on the robe, not quite sure how you wear something which is basically a sheet with some strings attached, and sat on the bed waiting.

In a few minutes the anesthesiologist came in and asked me to lie down and show him my backside.  I felt the sting of the needle in my thigh.  He said, "This is going to feel warm as I'm injecting it," and he wasn't kidding.  Whatever it was felt like liquid heat, and I could literally follow its path through my veins because as it traveled through me more and more body parts became warm and started to get a strange, tingling sensation to them.  Suddenly, I started to feel myself getting groggy and weaker.  When he returned in a few minutes, I felt oddly detached from my body and not quite sure I could get off the bed and onto the gurney, but I managed to do so and laid back as he pulled the sheet up onto me.  Then, I closed my eyes because it felt difficult to keep them open, and tried to take in as much as I could with my ears.

I heard the gurney softly rumbling through the hallway, heard the elevator door opening and closing twice as we traveled to the second floor, and then felt a slight lurch as the gurney stopped.  When I opened my eyes I could see that I was in some kind of prep room.  On another gurney in the room I saw a woman, not Anne, who I presumed was a non-transgender client in for some kind of plastic surgery or other.  The anesthesiologist picked up my limp left arm by the wrist and proceeded to lightly slap the back of the hand, looking for a place to insert an I.V. needle.  When he had it in place he left the room, and I closed my eyes again.  In a little while I felt the gurney start moving once more and, judging from the amount of light pouring in through my eyelids, we were soon in a very brightly lit room.  The gurney stopped amid the sounds of a number of people speaking in French, and in the background was the sound of a symphony playing lively, bright, classical music.

Opening my eyes, I saw a huge bank of about five lights hanging over me.  Each was like a big silver cone, and the five of them were arranged in a kind-of pentagon shape that was being supported by a heavy, green metal arm that came from the ceiling.  A post-op friend of mine had earlier (and aptly) described it to me as like looking up at the underside of a Saturn rocket.  I turned my head and saw Dr. Menard, my surgeon, standing nearby in his blue operation-room scrubs, a surgical cap on his head and his surgical mask hanging around his neck.  He smiled at me and waved.  I smiled and gave a weak wave back without saying anything.  Then I closed my eyes again, and that's all that I remember until I woke up.


## SO WHAT ACTUALLY HAPPENS DURING THIS OPERATION?

I give you fair warning that I'm going to be quite graphic in this part and use lots of words like: incision, penis, scrotum, urethra, clitoris, vagina, suture, and orange juice.  **Those of you who are squeamish about this kind of thing can easily pass over it all by skipping right to the part titled:  "OK ... YOU CAN OPEN YOUR EYES NOW."**

All right ... now ... while *I'm* safely tucked away in la-la land, and while the surgeon is working his magic on me to the strains of 'Bolero', or whatever the heck it is he's listening to, I think this would be a great time to tell you (as best I can) exactly what happens during the male-to-female surgery.  Put on your imagination caps because all *I* can provide is words; you're going to have to draw your own pictures.

Let's start with the position that the patient is placed in. Do a little experiment with yourself.  Stand up and spread your feet as far apart as you can get them.  Now, go into a squat as though you were trying to sit in a chair ... keep your back perpendicular to the floor.  Imagine yourself being frozen in this position and a couple of people come along and pick you up and lay you on your back on the operating table.  That's the position the patients are placed into after the anesthesiologist has done his thing and sent them into the stratosphere.

Next the surgical area is disinfected and the surgical draping (the cloths used to protect the parts of the body that are *not* going to be worked on) is put into place.

Now, a *big* needle ... I mean, in the video this needle looked like it was about six inches long ... is used to inject a solution into the scrotum, penile, and groin areas.  The solution deadens the nerves and causes the veins in the area to constrict so that blood loss is kept to a minimum.  Also, the surgeon uses a cauterizing scalpel for all incisions so that blood vessels are closed off as they are cut.  I was actually quite surprised to notice, while I was watching the video, how little blood loss occurs during this operation.

After the surgical areas are prepared in this way, several incisions are made.  The first one is made about one inch above the anus and is a small, semi-circular incision (about one inch in diameter) with its apex pointing towards the scrotum.  This small flap of skin in peeled outward (the lower part still attached to the body) and will later become part of the opening to the new vagina.  The second incision is made from the top of the first incision, up through the middle of the scrotum, and to the base of the penis.

This next part is where the orange juice comes in. We've all done this little trick when we have a can of frozen orange juice that we're in a hurry to use and we don't want to wait for it to thaw out. What we do is remove *both* ends of the can, then we take a knife and run it around the inside of the can (between the can and the frozen orange juice), and at that point we can use one of the can lids to push the frozen juice out of the can and into the pitcher. This is sort of what the surgeon does with the penis because what he wants is to have a tube of skin, still attached to the body and its blood supply, that can be turned inside-out to become the new vagina. So, after carefully removing the tip of the penis so as not to destroy the nerves that produce orgasm, he runs a surgical tool (kind of like a long, skinny, spatula) between the penile skin and the spongy, internal tissue of the penis. When this is done, he is able to pull the insides of the penis out of the skin tube from the bottom. It's really kind of slick.

Next, the testes and their sperm tubes are removed from the open scrotum, the tubes are sewn closed, cut, and the ends are allowed to retract into the body. That completes the castration.

Once that is done, the penile nerves (the ones which are responsible for producing orgasm) are carefully dissected from the skinless penis back to the point were they enter the torso. Then, the spongy penile tissue which surrounds the urethra is carefully cut (very close to the body) and removed, leaving just the urethral tube coming out of the torso.

At this point, the surgeon has a tube of skin (still attached to the body), an empty scrotal sac, a small bundle of nerve tissue, and a fairly long urethral tube that is coming out of the body.

Now, the penile nerves are shortened, and the remaining stump of nerves is laid in place against the body where it will become the new clitoris. The path of the urethra is altered so as to exit the body a little beneath the neo-clitoris and a catheter is inserted through the urethra and into the bladder.

Next, the new vaginal cavity is created.  The muscles located between the anus and the urethra (which in female-born people develop as a divided set of muscles surrounding the vaginal opening, but which in male-born people develop as a single, unbroken set of muscles) are slit in half lengthwise and separated to expose the internal tissues.  Working very carefully in order to avoid piercing the intestines, the bladder, the prostate, and whatever other organs are in the area, the surgeon cuts a pathway into the torso, between the intestines and the bladder, about two inches wide by five inches deep.

After that, the tube of penile skin is turned inside-out and, if necessary (and it almost always *is*), it is extended by taking what is now excess skin from the scrotum and sewing it into place at the end of the tube.  What used to be the skin on the outside of the penis is now on the inside of the tube and will become the walls of the new vagina, while the skin that used to be on the inside of the penis is now exposed and will end up in contact with the tissues in the torso (the penile and torso tissue eventually fusing together as they heal).  If you have a hard time visualizing this little maneuver, you can perhaps get a better idea of what it is like by grasping half of the rim of a sock (pretending that it is the empty tube of penile skin still attached to the body) and using your free hand to turn the sock inside-out.  You have just turned an "outtie" into an "innie"!

Before the new vaginal tube is inserted into the created body cavity, a small slit is cut into it at the point where it will pass over the neo-clitoris and the urethra, and the catheter tube is pulled through the slit.  This procedure ensures that both the clitoris and the urethral opening will be properly exposed and *not* completely covered over by skin, which would make it difficult to have sensation in the clitoris and impossible to pee.  What is now the vaginal tube is inserted into the vaginal cavity and positioned by sewing it to the flap of skin which was created with the very first incision that the surgeon made.

Things are now nearing an end.  The urethral tube, which now pokes out through the vulval skin, is still quite long, so (with the catheter still in place) it is shortened, the excess tissue removed, and the remaining, exposed urethral tube is slit along its length.  This leaves the surgeon with a little flap of mucous tube which is folded up to cover the clitoral nerves (providing them with both protection and a little lubrication) and sewn into place.

Next the soft, medical stent is inserted into the vagina and the vaginal opening is sewn partially closed to hold the stent in place.  The stent will remain where it is for the next six days, holding the vaginal tissue firmly against the internal tissues of the torso and allowing the two sets of tissue to begin fusing together as they heal.  The stent also prevents the body from effectively closing up the new vaginal cavity as it works to heal itself.

With all of that done, the remaining scrotal skin is folded back into place and sewn closed, creating the labia majora, and a dressing is sewn into place over the whole vulva area to help prevent bleeding and swelling.

Then, all the doctors and nurses and anesthesiologists clean up and go home to dinner with their loved ones while you are wheeled back into your room to begin your recovery.  C'est tout!!

Of course, there are other things which go on during this whole process but, hey, I'm not a doctor, and I wasn't looking while all of this was going on, so I explained it as best I could.

# OK ... YOU CAN OPEN YOUR EYES NOW.

**Surgery Day (continued):**

When I finally opened *my* eyes, it was for a very short time.  The next thing I remember after seeing Dr. Menard in the operation room was hearing the sounds of someone talking.  As I focused my mind I became aware that it was Anne, Cindy, and Barbara.  Cindy was asking how Anne was feeling, and Anne weakly replied, "Just tired, mostly, and there's quite a bit of pain." Then Barbara said something about that being usual and that it would decrease.  Anne asked what time it was and someone replied "Almost 6:00 p.m."  Then I opened my eyes just as Barbara looked over at me and she said, "Oh, Jean's awake!"

The two of them walked over to my bed ... I kind of remember their faces floating above me ... and Cindy asked, "How are you feeling?"  I thought for a moment and answered, "OK, I guess", but I don't remember saying anything else.

Barbara said, "Well, we just wanted to come make sure that ya'll were OK.  We've got to get back for supper, but I'll see you in a few days when you come back home."  Cindy added, "And I'll come back tomorrow to visit."  Then they said good-by and left.

The curtain was drawn between our beds, so I couldn't see Anne, but she spoke up and said, "Well, dear, we made it", to which I replied, "Ya, I guess we did."  Then I conked out again and don't remember anything until later that night ... much later that night ... when a nurse came in to check on us.

It turned out that this was only one of a regular schedule of visits that seemed to take place every few hours.  She took my pulse, temperature and blood pressure, and did something down in my groin area, though I couldn't tell what.  It felt like I'd been asleep *forever*, and I thought to myself, "It must be like three o'clock in the morning."  When I asked what time it was, she said,

"Eleven p.m.", and it was at that point that I realized the next few days were going to go *very* slowly.

As she was working I became aware that my mouth and throat felt unbelievably dry, and I asked for some water.  She responded that it was still too early for me to be drinking any-thing, so I assured her that I only wanted enough to wet my lips and throat.  She put a straw in my glass of water and held it to my lips saying, "Just a little."  I got two small sips before she pulled it away, and they were two of the most wonderful sips of water I think I've ever had.  When she was done she asked, "On a scale of one to ten, what would you say your pain is right now?"  I focused on my body for a few moments and replied, "Seven."  She nodded and left, returning in a few minutes with a needle of morphine which she put into my arm.  I closed my eyes and was asleep in no time.

**One Day After Surgery:**

The next morning I was woken up by two nurses who came in to do their nurse things to me.  Much of the anesthesia had worn off and I was actually alert enough to be aware of my surroundings and what was going on.  My pulse, temperature, and blood pressure were taken again.  Then they pulled down the blankets, lifted the johnny (all front, no back), and began to work in earnest.

I didn't bother to do more than lift my head, which did not exactly give me a good vantage point for seeing what was going on or how things looked, but that was OK since I really wasn't in the mood for being curious.  I could see that I was wearing some kind of surgical panty, something that looked very much like it was made of gauze but which stretched as though it were made of spandex or something.  The purpose of the panty seemed to be to hold various dressings and other medical stuff in place.

The first things to come out were two big ice packs, one from between my legs (right up by the crotch) and the other from on top of the pubic bone.  That gave me an idea of how little sensation I had in my groin area because I honestly had no idea before that moment that there were ice packs down there ... no sensation of cold whatsoever!

Next, the panty was pulled down and the top layer of gauze dressing was removed, showing me a large patch of very bruised and very swollen skin running from the upper part of the pubic bone to a little below the belly button and almost the whole width of my pelvis.  Below the external dressing was more dressing, sewn into place temporarily, which they inspected carefully but did nothing with.  Then one of the nurses brought out some kind of salve and began to anoint the area that was beyond my view, eventually working up to the upper edge of the pubic bone where I could just see a few sutures sticking up through the skin.  After that, a new external dressing went on and the panty was pulled back up.

Then came the "changing of the pad", a little procedure which I really came to appreciate as the day went on because it was the only chance I got (other than moving my feet, which we were often encouraged to do) to move my stiff, uncomfortable, and pained leg muscles.  "OK," they said, "now we need you to bend your legs up."  I did so, very slowly and painfully bringing my heels closer to my butt.  "That's fine," they said. "Now very easily lift your bottom up off the bed."  I braced my arms on the bed, put more weight onto my feet, and gingerly lifted my tush about two inches and held it there.  The nurses quickly slid the old gauze padding and plastic backing out from under me and slid a clean one into its place, letting me know that I could then settle back down again.

After that, one of the nurses went about changing the urine collection bag that was hanging at the foot of the bed and which was connected to me by a long plastic tube which disappeared somewhere under the gauze panty.

The nurse on my right turned to me, smiled, and asked if I'd like a back rub.  Well, she might as well have asked me if I wanted to go to heaven!  Yes, I wanted a back rub!  Every muscle in my back ached, and several places felt even more tender from lying on what seemed like particularly hard pieces of the bed.  "OK," she said, "I need you to roll over on your side.  Now go slowly!"  My left hand still had the IV feeding tube in it, so I couldn't move that one around much, but my right hand and arm were free, so I slowly reached over myself, grabbed the left bed-rail, and painfully pulled myself onto my left side.  She went to work right away, her hands coated with a wonderful soothing lotion, rubbing all the sore muscles and stimulating the circulation.  The pain eased a bit and I felt almost alive again, but all too soon it was over and she told me I could lie down on my back.

With all of that done, fresh ice packs were placed in my crotch area, the johnny was pulled down, and the blankets were pulled up and secured around me.  Then the same question was asked, "On a scale of one to ten, what would you say your pain level is right now?".  It was still "seven", and another shot of morphine went into my arm, after which I was left alone to nod back off to sleep ... or to wherever you go when you're full of morphine and your body is busy trying to heal itself.

This nursing procedure was repeated about every four hours or so, interspersed with naps, semi-consciousness, meal times, a visit from Anne's sister, Cindy, and very small talk with my room-mate in the other bed:

"Anne, is it raining out?"
"No."
"Jean, what time do you think it is?"
"I don't know.  Maybe about ten."
"Anne, are you in a lot of pain?"

"Yes ... are you?"
"Yes."
"I'm glad it's done."
A long pause. "Yeah, me too."

That day and night were *very* long, and very, very painful.  There didn't seem to be a muscle or joint anywhere in me
that didn't hurt in some way, and the situation was compounded
by the fact that we didn't have the energy to do a lot of moving
and really couldn't have if we wanted to because we were so
bundled up in blankets.  Every bump or fold in the mattress felt
like a little spike poking into me because I couldn't move enough
to relieve the pressure, and my muscles would scream from in-
activity and stiffness.  I often pushed the nurse-call button in order to have her change the positioning of the bed, and looking
back on it now I think that any relief came not from the final position but from the process of getting there, from being in motion if
only for a little while.
    Anne seemed to be having problems with hot flashes
and cold sweats (something which is quite common among new
MTF post-ops), and I had one or two of them myself.  First you're
trying to throw the blankets off because you're so hot you feel
like you're suffocating, then you're pulling them all back up
around you while the perspiration continues to flow, you feel like
you're freezing, and your teeth are chattering.
    Adding to my already less-than-rosy disposition was the
fact that I was feeling incredibly nauseous.  If I was lying flat on
my back, the nausea would subside enough to almost disappear;
but if the head of the bed was cranked up beyond maybe 30 degrees or so, my stomach would start doing somersaults and my
head would begin to spin.  This was not at all helpful when it
came time to eat.  The nurse would come in while I was lying flat
on my back (and actually feeling a little hungry) and take our

meal orders, then when the food got there and they raised my head so that I could eat ... I couldn't eat!

This posed a problem for the nursing staff because we really do need to be eating in order to begin regaining our strength.  Anne was eating fine (considering her condition), and was eating more substantial stuff with each meal.  I, on the other hand, was spurning all food.  Breakfast and lunch came and went and all I could get down was some cranberry juice.  The nurses were getting very concerned.

About mid-afternoon two of them came in to do the standard nursing procedure and for some reason ended up raising the head of my bed a bit too much.  "I'm sick!" I exclaimed ... "I'm going to throw up!"  They both took a step backwards in unison just as I somehow shot up into a sitting position and unloaded several cups of bile-and-whatever into the little plastic pan that they had brought in to hold the bandages they would be changing.  They glanced at each other as I sank back onto the bed, but rightly held their ground because a second later I somehow shot back up into the sitting position again and added another cup or so to the first load.  Then, truly exhausted, I fell back onto the pillow.  "I didn't know I could move that fast," I said weakly.

They stepped forward to clean things up and resume their job, and one of them, with a big smile on her face, said, "There!  Now you'll feel better!"  Well, actually, I *did* feel better, and we all had great hopes that I would now be able to eat, but when dinner time came it was the same old story.

Nevertheless, everyone encouraged me to eat.  Even Anne looked over from her bed and said, "Honey, you've got to eat *something*.  You need to get your energy back."

I thought, "Well, maybe the nausea right now is just the last bit left over from before and it's on its way out and will be gone a little later.  So, maybe if I make myself eat now it will actually help."

I picked up some of the food and put it into my mouth, chewing and swallowing it with great difficulty as my stomach did little swirls.  The nurses gave almost audible sighs of relief.  After several minutes of this procedure they decided that now that I was eating they could take out the IV feeding tube from my hand (Anne had had hers removed right after breakfast) and one of them came forward and finally gave freedom to my left arm.  But another few mouthfuls was all that I could handle, and I pushed the tray aside and lay back again.

A few hours later Dr. Menard came into the room to see how we were doing.  Anne gave her report which sounded pretty good to me, even though she talked about having quite a bit of pain, and then he turned to hear what I had to say.  I told him about my nausea and how it would only manifest if I was sitting up.  Then I told him how I had a similar experience years before when I had all four of my wisdom teeth removed at the same time and how we had finally figured out that I was reacting to the medication rather than the pain.  He agreed that it was possible and said that he would prescribe a different pain killer for me to see how that would work.  Then he turned to the nurse with him and said, "We should put her back on the IV, huh, until we have this fixed and we know she's eating."

After he left I watched in horror as the nurse approached me and proceeded to reinstall the IV feeding tube into my RIGHT hand!  I thought to myself, "Wait a minute.  That's my RIGHT hand!  That's the one that reaches my water glass!  That's the one that pushes the nurse-call button!  If I can't move *that* hand around I'm going to be totally helpless!!"  But, for some unknown reason, I kept my mouth shut and only managed to request that the nurse-call button be repositioned so that I could at least reach it with my left hand.

Then I was alone and feeling pretty miserable.  Anne was in and out of sleep, as was I, and neither of us was exactly a fountain of conversation when we were awake, so I had plenty of time to just lie there and think.  I distinctly remember thinking, "OK, Jean, tell me again ... *why* did you do this?"  I knew why I had done it, and there was *never* any doubt that it was the right thing to do, but lying in that bed at that moment it seemed like a good question to be asking.

Later that evening, when the next round of nursing procedure was finishing up and the nurse approached me with the syringe, I held up my left hand and said, "Wait a minute.  Is that morphine?."

"No, no," she replied, "The doctor changed your prescription to something else," at which point I signaled her to let me have it.

For some reason, night time seemed to amplify the pain and discomfort.  Maybe it was because the hubbub and sounds of the daytime slowed down and disappeared, leaving me with nothing else to focus on except my body and how it was feeling.  At any rate, Wednesday night was *very* rough.  My muscles stiffened, the bed-sores seemed worse, the nausea continued, and I was hot and wanted nothing more than a cooling breath of fresh outdoor air rather than the stale, recirculated, hospital air.  I took the sleeping pills that were offered, but they really didn't do anything, and the only thing that helped was to get a pain shot as often as they would give them to me and then nod off for an hour or two.  The night seemed eternal, and every waking moment in it had some kind of pain.

**Two Days After Surgery:**

Nevertheless, at some time during the night a little threshold seemed to have been passed and the nauseating grip that the morphine had on me finally disappeared as it worked its way out of my system and the new pain-killer took over.

The nursing procedure also continued through the night at regular intervals, which provided me with a little bit of mental diversion from the overall aching that was going on during my awake time.

As the sun started coming up, more things began to happen.  Breakfast was served right around 7:00 am, and I was happy to discover that with the nausea gone I was actually able to eat some solid food and even had an appetite for it.  My breakfast that morning was mostly liquid and easily digested items: toast, cereal, sherbet, camomile tea, and juice.

Dr. Brassard came in shortly after that and quickly removed the layer of packing gauze that had been sewn into place over the surgical site.  I didn't bother to watch the procedure much because I figured that my point-of-view wasn't going to allow me to see a lot anyway.  The sutures were snipped with some scissors and pulled out, the gauze packing was lifted off and dumped into a disposal container, and the nurses did a quick sponging of the area with some kind of antiseptic liquid.  Then, because I had finally eaten, the IV feeding tube was removed from my right hand, freeing that up as well.

Now that the gauze packing was gone, Anne and I were allowed to get up and walk around a bit.  We would sit up very slowly in bed, swing our legs around to the side and, with a nurse holding on to us lest our legs give out underneath us, we would kind of slide off the bed into a standing position, simultaneously sticking our feet into our slippers.  Absolutely no bending over was allowed.  If something dropped to the floor, a nurse would have to retrieve it for us.  When no nurse was around we became creative, learning how to pick things up with our toes and delivering them to our hands by bending only our lower leg.

Stiff, immobilized joints got back into action and immediately began to feel much better.  Unfortunately, while the overall pain lessened considerably, it didn't completely go away.  There was always a dull ache somewhere in the background.  In addition, a new pain began to emerge in the groin area.  It was now about 48 hours after surgery and the nervous system down there was finally starting to come out of shock and regain some sensation.  As long as I was lying in bed or not moving around much, it was almost unnoticeable, but as soon as I started moving about and walking the pain would become quite enlivened.  So, it was a bit of a trade-off.  When I would lie still my groin would feel OK but the rest of me would hurt and feel uncomfortable.  When I got up and moved around to exercise my muscles, the rest of me would feel great but my groin would hurt.  Nevertheless, it was variety, and it was variety that I could choose and control, so things definitely seemed to be getting better.

We were encouraged to take a shower.  I went first, and standing in front of the mirror in the bathroom was the first opportunity for me to actually *see* how the surgery looked.  It wasn't pretty.  Almost everything was some shade of black, blue, deep maroon, or yellow from a little below my belly button right down into the top of my thighs and continuing between my legs and onto my butt.  The whole groin area was swollen considerably.  The suture lines running up the labia majora were very obvious, as were a variety of other sutures here and there, and down below I could just make out the surgical stent trying to force its way out of the new vagina and past the sutures which were holding it in place.  Then, hanging down amidst it all was the bright-yellow plastic tubing of the catheter, one end disappearing into the swollen "me" and the other end plugged with a white plastic stopper.  Strangely enough, though, I wasn't upset by the sight.  There was no scrotum, and there was no penis, and in amongst the swollen and discolored flesh I could still make out the definite promise of a new, decidedly feminine form, and I was thrilled!

I stood there for several minutes, inspecting myself in the mirror and gently touching various areas.  Then I pulled myself away and got into the shower ... a wonderfully warm, soft, relaxing shower.  I washed my hair for the first time in four days and gently massaged all my aching muscles as I washed.  It was heaven!

After getting out of the shower and drying off, I discovered that I had to urinate but, with the catheter still in place, the only way I could do that was standing up!  I hadn't stood up to urinate in almost two years!  I have to admit, I found it a little psychologically difficult to do.  Here I was with this new female form and the only way that I could pee was by acting like a guy!  But, it was obvious that my bladder needed to be emptied, so I had no choice.  I stood over the toilet, feeling very self-conscious, grabbed the end of the plastic tube, pinched it closed, and pulled out the little white plug.  Then I lowered my hand to hold the end of the tube over the middle of the toilet and un-pinched it.  A stream of urine came slowly running out (I was doing absolutely nothing to force or encourage it) and after about 15 or 20 seconds it slowed and stopped, followed by a quick little twinging sensation in my bladder which I took as the sign that the process was done.  I put the little white stopper back into the tube, disinfected the toilet seat in preparation for the next person, and went about drying and combing my hair.  Then I put on my robe and returned to the room.

With food, a little more of my energy had returned, and with more energy and more motion time seemed somehow to go more quickly.

Anne and I spent more time talking together, comparing notes about how we were feeling and what we remembered, trying to keep track in our minds of what everyone else must be doing back at the residence, excitedly speculating about what our future lives might be like, and trying to decide which parts of us would become *what* once the swelling had gone down.

Anne's sister, Cindy came by to visit for a last time before she had to fly back home, and when the visit was over Anne walked her to the lobby door so that the two of them could chat a bit alone.  On her return to the room, Anne settled back into bed and was quiet for a while before saying, "I'm going to miss seeing her."

"I can understand that," I replied.  "She's really a wonderful lady."

"She really *is* a wonderful lady," Anne said, nodding. "I
love her a lot.  It really meant so much to me to have her here."

"Maybe you ought to try to see her more often than once
every five years," I suggested.

"Yes ... I'm definitely going to try," she answered.

After that, I settled in to take a nap, the first of several,
comfortable naps that I would have during the day and which I
apparently needed to help make up for lost sleep the previous
nights.

I must have slept for an hour or two, but it seemed like
almost immediately that the nurse was back in our room asking
what we would like for lunch.  My appetite had definitely increased since breakfast, but I resisted ordering everything on the
menu and managed to keep my food intake moderately light,
mostly because I remembered what Phillippa had gone through
as a result of eating too much before her digestive system had
gotten back into gear.  Breakfast had been the first meal with
anything solid in it that I had had in four days, my stomach was
making no rumbling sounds, and I had definitely *not* had a bowel
movement.  After cleaning my plate and having raspberry sherbet for dessert, Anne and I chatted for a bit longer, then I did a
little bit of walking around to loosen my muscles again and laid
back to take another nap.

It really was a very nice nap.  Now that I could move
about, I began to experiment with finding a variety of comfortable
positions that I could lie in.  Each one had its pros and cons.  A
particular set of muscles would become relaxed while another
set would become stiffer, and intermixed with muscle comfort
was varying degrees of groin pain.  The most consistently restful
position (the one that I could stay in for the longest time with the
least amount of stiffness or pain) was lying on my side with a
pillow between my legs.  There was something about that pillow

between my legs that just made everything seem easier and more comfortable.  I don't know why it worked, but it did.  When I mentioned the arrangement to Anne she tried it too and got the same results.  For the next six weeks I would be sleeping with a pillow between my legs ... it took that long before I felt comfortable without it.

The nursing procedure was continuing at regular intervals through all of this, but once the bandages had been taken off it had been altered slightly to include only pulse, temperature, blood pressure, and a back rub.  My response to the "On a scale of one to ten..." question had gone from "seven" down to "five" by Thursday morning and had worked itself down even further during the day so that by nine or ten o'-clock that evening it was down to "between three and four", as which point the injections were stopped and we were given our pain-killers in pill form instead.

Another nap, and before long it was time for dinner.  My appetite was still increasing, and I had an even larger meal that night, though I resisted any kind of second helpings.  Before going to bed we also each got a pill to help soften our stools, making it easier (it was hoped) to have a bowel movement.  It was clear that the nursing staff wanted to see us use the bathroom for something other than showering and admiring our swollenness in the mirror.

As usual, with the nighttime came a big decrease in all activity and diversions and a proportionate increase in physical pain and discomfort.  Even though the aches were still big enough to make it difficult to sleep, the pain was clearly nothing compared to what it had been like the previous two nights.  Plus, I now had the ability to move about if any position became unbearable, and I took lots of advantage of that.  I would sleep for a couple of hours and then, when I became too uncomfortable, I would push the nurse-call button.  When she came into the room I would look at her pleadingly and ask, "May I go for a walk?  I need to loosen my muscles."  She always told me I could, and I would get up, put on my bathrobe and slippers, slip my arm into hers, and be escorted for one or two laps around the nurse's station and back into the room where I would sleep for another couple of hours before repeating the process.  She was really very kind and never showed any kind of impatience with my repeated, nocturnal promenades.  In this way I got through the night with more rest than I had gotten the previous two nights.

## RECUPERATION AT THE 'RESIDENCE'


**Three Days After Surgery:**

This was the day that we went back to the residence, so a good deal of our psychological attention was spent preparing for that.

The nursing procedure was cut back further so that now the nurses were helping us only if we needed something specific and were dispensing pain pills as we needed them.  Pulse, blood pressure, and temperature were no longer taken.  For the most part Anne and I were able to take care of ourselves.  We were still not allowed to bend over and would not do it even if it was allowed because there was still a lot of pain associated with large movements of the waist and lower body.  If something needed to be retrieved that was too heavy to pick up with our toes, the procedure was to slowly get down onto our knees (being careful to bend at the waist as little as possible) and then to lean over sideways enough to reach it.  The combination of the pain pills and the fact that some parts of the body were still a little in shock, and thus insensitive, worked well to hold the pain in check.

My appetite continued to improve and I was now eating full, honest-to-goodness meals.  After breakfast I decided that another shower would be in order because the one I took the day before felt so good.

Soon after the shower came a bowel movement, my first in four days.  Many of the abdominal muscles were still a bit dazed and weak, and trying to force the stools out would be quite painful because of all the stitches in the area, so the procedure became one of simply sitting and waiting for gravity to do its work.  This turned out to be the longest and most sensuous bowel movement I have ever had in my life!  It was also a psychological relief of sorts because I now knew that the stomach was working OK.  When I was done I wiped, then turned on the bidet to wash the area, then wiped again, then disinfected the toilet seat for the next person.  It was a process that was going to be repeated every time I used the toilet for the next six weeks, and it certainly made using the bathroom something of a production number.

Anne and I spent most of the morning chatting and napping.  Claudia and Phillippa were through with their stays at the residence and had been released to return home.  The tradition in Montreal is for released post-ops on their way out of town to stop by the clinic to see how the new post-ops are doing and to offer any final words of advice about what can be expected during the next week, so Phillippa and Claudia both paid us a call.  They were doing well, their dilations were going fairly smoothly, and they offered us some thoughts and encouragement on handling pain.

After lunch, we set about packing things up and getting dressed for the trip back to the residence.  There really was very little need to get dressed since we would spend a total of about 60 seconds walking from the back door of the clinic into the waiting van and then, after a four-minute drive, another 60 seconds walking from the van into the residence ... not much time to be seen by the general public, and a simple bathrobe and a blanket would have been fine to keep us from getting cold.  Subjectively, however, there was something about being dressed for the first time in four days that felt good.  It was like a milestone of sorts, an indication that we were moving closer to being on our own with our new bodies, and a reassurance that for all we had been through so far we were still capable of taking care of ourselves.  I think it was also important, at least to me, to be able to walk into the residence with my psychological "chin" up as an encouragement for the pre-ops who would be there when we returned.  Anne and I didn't know them yet, but they would soon be going through the same pain and discomforts that we'd been through, and it seemed important that they at least have the impression that it was something that one could survive.

An hour or so after lunch, a van showed up to take us back to the residence.  After saying good-bye to the nurses and thanking them for all their help and care, Anne and I got into the back and gingerly sat on the pillows that had been provided.  It was a nice, sunny day, and it was wonderful to be seeing green grass and people, feeling the cool breeze, and breathing in the fresh outdoor air.  We were going home, and we had actually come to think of the residence as just that ... home.

When the short ride was over, we climbed out of the van and walked slowly into the house where Marie-Andree, Raphael, Lee, and Barbara (all familiar faces) were waiting to greet us.  Hugs and smiles went all around, and everyone remarked on how "good" (i.e. healthy) we looked.  The new group of pre-ops were also there, and we all stood in the living room for a few minutes meeting each other and exchanging pithy informational sound-bites such as: "Don't worry, you'll be fine"...."This is really the experience of a lifetime"....and "Oh, God, the nurses over there are all *angels*!"  There would be plenty of time over the next few days to answer people's deeper questions.

The pre-ops (and their significant others) for the following week consisted of: Beverly (an MTF in her late forties) and her wife, Donna;  Vicky (a 21 year-old MTF) and her mother, Susan; and Joan (a 25 year-old MTF).  Beverly and Vicky would have their surgery on Monday; Joan would have her's on Tuesday.

Marie-Andree informed us that all our suitcases had been placed in the upstairs back room, and after a few more minutes of chatting we excused ourselves in order to unpack and rest before supper time.

So far we hadn't exerted ourselves very much, so we still had enough energy to unpack our suitcases and set up our room the way we wanted it.  Unfortunately, we were also not very mobile, which caused the process to take an hour or two.  The first thing to do was to take note of all the flowers and cards that our friends and families had sent to us while we were in the clinic.  There must have been six or eight bouquets of flowers between the two of us, and I also had half-a-dozen cards.  I read each of my cards and looked at and smelled each of the bouquets.  Then I turned to Anne and asked her *where* we were going to put them all.  There was a little space available on the headboards of our beds, we each had a small nightstand, and there was a third, unused bed in the room with its own headboard and nightstand, but other than that there was really no place to put all the vases, and we needed the area around our beds for the medical supplies we would be using.  After some thought we put two of the vases on the third headboard, Anne kept one of her bouquets on her headboard, and I went around the house discreetly dropping off vases of flowers on mantles, coffee tables and shelves.

In each of the nightstands were a number of under-pads, large squares of gauze with plastic backing which we were asked to keep under our butts while sleeping and, later, dilating.  There was still a moderate amount of discharge fluid (and sometimes small amounts of blood) coming from our surgery sites, and it was not uncommon for it to soak through our white cotton panties while we slept.  The pads were intended to protect the sheets and mattresses beneath us.

Each nightstand also had a couple boxes of panty liners, and we went through those like they were candy.  For the next week we would be replacing them, on average, about once every three hours.

Lubricating jelly, a mirror, antibiotic creme, the container with three stents, a water glass, a disposable douche, and a few other small items went on the top of the nightstand and within easy reach of the bed.  Combs, brushes, toothbrush, toothpaste, shampoo, extra lubricating jelly and antibiotic creme, a razor, and other toiletries went in the drawer.

On the headboards we had medications, the reading lamps, facial tissues, paper towels, our radios, and whatever else we had room for.  The one clock-radio in the room was placed on the third bed where we could both see the time.

A few of our clothes and things were left in our suitcases because it seemed unlikely we would be needing them, and the rest were placed in the three small drawers which were located under each of our beds.

A little while after we began this whole process, Marie-Andree came into the room to ask us how we were doing with pain and to ask if either of us needed a pain pill.  We had a choice of "regular or strong", and we both opted for a strong one which she dutifully retrieved from their locked storage cabinet in the office.  She also brought each of us another stool-softener pill and made sure that we knew we could have those whenever we felt we needed them.  Thus we were reminded, although we had known it from Phillippa's experience, that at this stage of the game everyone was going to be very interested in seeing that our digestive tracts were properly re-activated and busy at work. I took both of my pills right away.

We were also each issued one of the famous rubber donuts that each post-op gets.  These things look like miniature tire
inner tubes, usually bright red, and are intended to be inflated
and sat upon, the thought being that they will make sitting more
comfortable.  Well, sometimes they *do* make it easier to sit,
sometimes they don't.  Sometimes they need to be inflated more,
sometimes they need to be deflated a bit to be softer.  At all
times they need to be used in combination with one or more pillows, and it usually takes several attempts to find just the right
combination for a particular chair ... it all depends on the individual and how that person is feeling on any given hour of the day.
About the best they were actually able to do was to make sitting
bearable but still very uncomfortable.  Together with the one or
two pillows that we each carried around with us for the next six
days, the rubber donuts comprised our chair survival kit, were
used often, and were sworn at frequently.

After getting unpacked and set up in our new bedroom,
Anne and I chatted a bit more and then lay down for yet another
nap.

For dinner we showed up just as we had seen Claudia
and Phillippa do a week earlier, two pillows and rubber donut in
hand.  Lee still had his place of honor at the head of the table
and I chose to sit near him in order to have a little more room to
negotiate into and out of the chair with.  I think it took about three
tries to find a position that would let me sit long enough to eat.
The talk at dinner was about many things but was largely divided
into the categories of "pre-ops telling about themselves" and
"post-ops telling about the clinic experience".  Most of the questions aimed at Anne and me were about what would happen at
the clinic and how folks could expect to feel after surgery.  We
really didn't pull any punches and made sure that they knew it
was going to be painful.  Beverly (in her late 40's) kind-of
brushed it off, and Vicky (21 years-old) seemed very concerned
and freely admitted to having a low pain threshold.  Lee, Anne,

and I all tried to reassure her and her mother, Susan, that it was not something that she couldn't get through and that the morphine would take the sharpest edges off of the pain.  Nevertheless, she was clearly a little shaken by it because she had, for some reason, thought that the whole procedure would be relatively painless.

Back in our room after supper, Anne and I asked each other if we should have been as explicit as we were, but after talking about it for a while we decided that, *yes*, we should have been and that it was more helpful for Vicky to know ahead of time and be able to psychologically prepare herself than to be completely surprised when she woke up after surgery.  It was also good for her mother, who was going to be with Vicky and supporting her, to know what to expect in order to be better able to help.

After lounging in our room for a while, Anne decided to visit with everyone else in the living room for a short time before going to bed.  I decided to just go to bed after getting a glass of juice from the kitchen.  On my way to the kitchen I ran into Marie-Andree who looked at me very seriously and asked, "Have you had a bowel movement yet?"  Well, as a matter of fact, I had made a number of trips to the bathroom throughout the afternoon and so I looked at her and said, "Yes, I've had three bowel movements."

She looked at me with surprise on her face and asked, "You've had three bowel movements since yesterday?!"

"No," I replied, "I've had three bowel movements in the last five hours!"

A little grin appeared on her face and she shook her finger at me and said, with mock sternness, "No more pills for you!"  Then, after a pause, she added, "You're doing OK ... you're going to be fine."

I went to bed, pillow between my legs, and slept in little blocks of two or three hours interspersed with being awake for

an hour or so in between each block.  This was pretty much the
sleeping schedule that I would have for several more weeks.
During my waking time I would reach for my little radio, put on
the earphones, and see what I could pick up for background music while I lay in bed thinking and waiting to fall asleep again.
This procedure of through-the-night radio listening went on almost every night for the remainder of my stay in Montreal, and I
really found it quite interesting.  It was impossible to find an
English-speaking station playing american top-40's, so I would
surf the dial, listening to French, Chinese, Pakistani, and Middle-
Eastern speaking stations and music.  At one point (about 2:00
AM) I noticed that Anne was awake as well and I suggested that
she tune in to the station I was listening to, a station that was
playing something that sounded like middle-east islamic music
but which the musicians were obviously improvising on in an almost jazz-like manner.  She found it, listened for a short time,
and then announced: "Oh, yeah, that's called Moroccan-roll.
Nice stuff!"

     We each listened for a while and then took off the head-
sets and chatted a bit.  Anne was having problems with hot
flashes, a *very* common problem for post-ops who have suddenly lost most of their testosterone supply but who are not yet
back on estrogens ... it's kind of like going through menopause.
Every post-op I've talked with has experienced these hot flashes
during the days between surgery and restarting estrogen, some
just a little (as in my case) others very heavily (going through five
or six sets of sheets in a night as a result of all their perspiring).
Personally, I think that there is a correlation between the pre-
surgery dosage of estrogen that someone is taking and the
amount of trouble they are likely to have with hot flashes ...
higher levels of pre-surgery estrogen resulting in more and
stronger hot flashes ... but I have no way of proving that.  All I
know is that my doctor had me on fairly low levels of estrogen,

compared to other transsexuals I have known, and my problems
with hot flashes were almost non-existent.

Another experience which most post-ops have, but
which also seems to vary widely from person to person, is what
is referred to among the initiates as "electric shocks".  The doctors tell us that what feels like quick, mild, random, internal, electric jolts in the surgical area are the result of nerve endings growing back together and re-establishing themselves after surgery.
I've never heard of anyone being incapacitated by these jolts
(which can literally come at any time of the night or day and may
last from a quick millisecond to a second or two), but they can
certainly be strong enough to cause the person to visibly flinch.
Most of the shocking comes during the first two or three weeks
after surgery and then becomes less frequent.  In my case, I had
a few "shocks", all very quick and slight, during the first two
weeks after surgery and then almost none after that.  Nevertheless, I *was* still getting them as much as two or three months afterwards.


**Four Days After Surgery:**


Something new happens for a change ... I have a day
that is totally unremarkable!!  I get up when I wake up, wash, eat,
rest, talk, sleep some more, read a little, and don't even bother to
try dressing, spending the entire day in my night gown, robe, and
slippers.  The overall body aches and pains subside noticeably
(which makes some things easier and more pleasant to do), but
they begin to be replaced by localized pain and soreness in the
surgical area as that part of my body continues to wake up.

Anne and I spend a good deal of time chatting with Lee
and Barbara and the pre-op folks.  I am impressed by the kind of
quiet, spiritual strength that Lee and Barbara have continued to
show throughout his ordeal and the patience and compassion
that both he and Barbara have tried to show to each other and to

the other folks around them.  Lee assures me that he has no
desire to be politically active or publicly "out" in any way: "I just
want to go home, and mow my lawn, and lead a quiet life."  Still,
when I talk with Anne about him, I find that she has the same
impressions and we both agree that, even if he only decides to
work quietly, one-on-one, without being public about it, he will
still be a very spiritually powerful brother for other trans men as
they work on their own transitions.

## Five Days After Surgery:

I guess I should have known.  One day of relative calm
and lessening pain shouldn't lead me to believe that I am out of
the woods yet.

What was a fairly small pain in the crotch area on Saturday has increased considerably overnight as the area continues
to "wake up" and discover that something isn't quite the way it
remembers.  The muscles on either side of the opening to the
new vagina, which used to be one group of muscles and which
were slit lengthwise in order to make the opening, are now as
hard as rock and don't want to move at all.  In addition, the
medical stent within the new vagina is straining on the sutures
that are holding it in place, creating a pulling force on the skin
and muscles that the sutures pass through (in the same way that
a foot might strain against the shoelaces of an under-sized shoe
that it has been forced into).  The unyielding muscles and pulling
sutures, combined, mean that any movement or pressure on the
area, like walking or sitting, brings immediate jolts of pain and a
sensation similar to having pins stuck into your skin.  It doesn't
take me long to figure out that no motion is good motion.

I spend all of Sunday and Sunday night trying to move
as little as possible and take to either sitting in one of the reclining lounge chairs (so that my body weight is transferred to my
back rather than my butt) or lying in bed (napping or reading).  I

also take the maximum number of pain pills that the staff will let me have.  At meal times I stand at the counter to eat.  I know from Claudia's and Phillippa's experience that this latest little episode will only last for a day and that one of the surgeons will come by the residence the next morning to remove the stent and catheter and give us freedom.  That knowledge provides some solace ... but it is not a great day.

This is also the day that Beverly and Vicky leave for the clinic as their surgeries are scheduled for the next morning. Joan, whose surgery is Tuesday morning, will not head for the clinic until Monday evening.  At dinner there is a lot of subdued conversation.  Beverly seems to be doing OK with preparing herself psychologically, but Vicky is clearly worried about the pain. Lee, Barbara, Anne, and I do what we can to reassure her that everything will be OK, that the nurses at the clinic will take very good care of her, and that whatever pain she might experience will *not* be something that she won't be able to make it through.  I really can't tell whether our words make any difference to her, but then I also realize that it's impossible to convey to someone else beforehand what a subjective experience, like pain, is going to be like.  She's just going to have to go through it, like we did, and like everyone else who has ever had the surgery has had to.  We can empathize, but we can't take the experience away from her.

After dinner, Beverly and Vicky finish their packing and head for the clinic amid hugs and good-byes and a promise from Anne and I that we will come visit them before we leave on Friday morning.  Donna goes with Beverly and Susan with Vicky to help them get settled in, leaving Lee, Barbara, Anne, Joan, myself, and a few staff people to chat for a while in the living room. I finally get tired enough and head for bed and another night of two-hour sleeping blocks and listening to Moroccan-roll.

**Six Days After Surgery:**

Dr. Brassard arrived at 6:30 a.m. with Sylvia to remove our stents and catheters.  The early hour was not a problem for Anne or me as we were both wide awake and had already done a bit of cleaning up in the bathroom in anticipation of the event. When they knocked on the door and came into our bedroom, they found Anne and me lying on our respective beds, naked from the waist down, impatiently waiting.  Our eagerness to have the stents and catheters out must have been apparent in our faces because Dr. Brassard grinned a little and asked, "Are you two ready?"

"Oh, yes," we replied, "we're very ready!  Let's do it!" Sylvia moved a portable folding screen to between the beds so that we couldn't see what was happening with each other (don't ask me why she did that ... it didn't matter to either of us whether we saw the other person or not ... but she did it anyway).  Anne was first, and in less than a minute she was saying, "Oh, wow, that feels much better!"  Then I heard Dr. Brassard say, "OK, now we take out the catheter", followed by a little exclamation from Anne, and her procedure was over.

Now it was my turn.  They came around the screen, he pulling on a fresh pair of examination gloves, Sylvia standing by with a disposable container for the medical supplies.  I spread my legs and closed my eyes, not particularly caring to see what was going to come out from inside me.  "OK", he said, "we start by snipping the sutures", and as he snipped I could feel the tension on the crotch muscles release in little stages.  Then the medical stent slid out very easily and painlessly, and I heard him deposit it in the container that Sylvia held nearby.  Then, suddenly, I felt a twinge and a warm feeling in the urethra (very like the sensation one feels just as you start to urinate) and I thought to myself, "Oh, no ... I'm going to pee on the bed!"  Just as I finished thinking that he said, "Now I'm removing the catheter," and

as he finished making that statement the sensation went away.
"There, all done," he said.  I noticed right away that the pain and
stinging sensation was gone completely (replaced by a low-level,
dull, discomfort from the swollen area) and that I felt *much* better.
The whole procedure had taken a total of about four minutes for
the both of us.

Sylvia moved the screen back to its place by the door
and Dr. Brassard promised to come back the next day to see
how we were doing.  Then, after telling us that Sylvia would next
be instructing us in how to dilate and douche, he left, heading for
the clinic where he was scheduled to operate on Beverly about
an hour later.

Let me digress here to explain "dilating" a little bit.
When male-to-female sexual reassignment surgery (SRS) is finished, the patient ends up with a soft, medical stent sewn inside
the new vagina.  The stent is kind of like a soft dildo, a penis-
shaped object.  The purpose of the stent is twofold: first (because the vagina is not sewn into place internally) to hold the
internal skin of the vagina firmly against the surrounding tissue
so that it can heal and adhere to the tissue; and second, to hold
the vagina open against the pressure of the surrounding tissue
and muscles.  Those who have had their ears pierced know that
after the piercing is done it's necessary to keep a stud of some
kind in the hole long enough for the skin to heal around it, otherwise the newly-pierced hole will simply heal closed.  Well, in a
sense, the new vagina is kind of like a giant piercing, and the first
impulse of the body is to try to heal this new opening closed.
The way it is prevented from healing closed is by keeping some
kind of stud (called a "dilator" or "stent") inside the vagina while it
is healing.

As it happens, complete healing of the vagina can take
six months to a year, and even after that the body will still be trying to slowly close things up.  Happily, post-op MTF transsexuals
do not have to keep a dilator inside themselves 24 hours a day

for six to twelve months.  It has been found, through trial and error over the years I am sure, that inserting a dilator into the new vagina and leaving it there for a period of time, and repeating that process at regular intervals during the day, is enough to get the body used to the idea that the new way that things are is the way that things should be.

This process of inserting a stent into the new vagina is called "dilating".  When a newly post-op transsexual first begins dilating, it needs to be done fairly frequently.  As healing continues over the following weeks and months, the number of dilations per day are slowly reduced until the post-op transsexual is finally dilating perhaps once or twice a week.  Experience has shown that once or twice a week is about as infrequently as dilations can be done in order to keep the vagina from closing up, and the new transsexual woman will have to dilate at least once or twice a week for the rest of her life.

The dilators, which we were asked to purchase before we arrived in Montreal, come in a set of five, all the same length but of varying diameters (from 1 inch to 1 1/2 inches in 1/8 inch increments).  They are made of a hard medical plastic, look and feel somewhat like ivory, are eight inches long, and one end of each of them is smoothly rounded like the skinny end of an egg. Of the five dilators in the set, the largest and smallest ones are not used, only the middle three, which most post-ops quickly learn to refer to as #1, #2, and #3.  A few folks, feeling more playful, may choose to name each of their dilators.  So ... with this understanding, we can get back to Sylvia.

Sylvia then explained the dilating process to us.  It was really quite straightforward.

***   Run a shallow, luke-warm bath (using anti-bacterial soap) and soak the surgical area for about five minutes to both clean and soften it.

***   Return to our room where we each have the three dilators in the container next to each of each of our beds.  All of the dilators have had a black ring drawn around them five inches from the tip, and all have been numbered according to their diameters.

***   Set out one of the protective gauze/plastic pads, placing it under our butt, and gather around us our three dilators, KY-jelly, paper towels, toilet paper, and a small mirror.

***   Starting with the smallest stent, #1, take it from the container of anti-bacterial solution that it is stored in, wipe if off with a paper towel, apply sterile KY-jelly from the tube to the first two or three inches of the tip (being careful not to touch it with our fingers),and then (using the mirror to see where we're going) insert the dilator into the vaginal opening and slowly push it into the vagina as close as we can get to the 5-inch mark.  (Simultaneously, we should be keeping the dilator as close to parallel with the bed as possible, *not* pointing down, to avoid the possibility of puncturing the vaginal and rectal walls which are now very close to each other).

***   Once the #1 stent has been in place for three minutes, remove it and place it aside on a paper towel and repeat the same procedure for the #2 stent.

***   Once the #2 stent has been in place for five minutes, remove it and place it with the #1 stent and repeat the same procedure for the #3 stent.  The #3 stent is supposed to be in place for 25 minutes, but the actual length of time for each stent is somewhat flexible.  The idea is to get the #3 stent into place and keep it there for a good length of time during each dilation session.

***   When done with the #3 stent, remove it and place it with the others, use toilet paper to clean up a bit, and then go into the bathroom and use the bidet to finish cleaning the area.

***   Wash the stents with disinfectant soap before returning them to their anti-bacterial storage bath.


After giving us all of this instruction, Sylvia left us to do our first session, saying that she would be in the kitchen (which was within earshot) if we needed help or had questions.  She also told us to let her know when we were done and she would show us how to douche as part of the cleanup.

Anne and I went to work (using the 3-5-25 minute schedule), asking each other questions and comparing experiences as we were proceeding.  The #1 and #2 stents gave only minimal discomfort and we had no problem inserting them the full five inches.  But when we came to the #3 stent we both kind of looked at each other, questioning whether something that large would actually fit where it was supposed to go.  Well, it did fit, but not very easily, and the sore, hard muscles on each side of the new vaginal opening did their uncomfortable best to stay tight enough to keep the stent out.  When the 25 minutes were up and we slowly removed the #3 stent we both felt our bodies relax noticeably and realized that over the 25 minutes it had been in there most of our body muscles had tightened up in reaction to the discomfort it was creating.  I had heard that, at first, getting the dilators up to the five-inch mark might take a number of minutes and might involve a certain amount of discomfort (translate that as "pain"), but that as the muscles in the area loosen up and begin to learn what is expected of them the whole process is easier, less painful, and goes more quickly.  I have also heard someone describe the dilating process for new, post-op, transsexuals as being something akin to impaling yourself.  Well, it's not that bad, but it's definitely a strain on various muscles, on the overall physiology, and even on the psyche, and most folks find it to be a very physically tiring exercise even though the whole thing is done while lying on your back.  Still, we were done with it, and we assumed that as we dilated more and more the whole process would become easier, so we said little about it.  We cleaned up a bit and then told Sylvia that we were ready for her.

It is common for the inside of the new vagina to slough off dead skin and some scar tissue for a number of weeks after surgery, so Sylvia joined us in the bathroom and instructed us on how to douche in order to flush those out.  We were told to douche at least twice a day, but for my own peace of mind (and with Sylvia's OK) I decided to douche each time I dilated.

The whole procedure (soaking, setting up, dilating, cleaning, and douching) took a little more than an hour, and for the rest of the time that we were at the residence we did these dilation sessions five times a day....which meant a total of about six hours a day doing medical maintenance.  It was suggested to us that we do one session before breakfast, one session before lunch, two sessions between lunch and dinner, and a final session immediately after dinner ... all of which sounded acceptable to us.

One thing which we experienced very soon after the catheters were removed was the new sensation of peeing while sitting *without* having the old ability to control where the urine stream would be going.  For newly post-op MTFs this lack of control is enhanced by the fact that the urethra has been dilated by the catheter, re-routed somewhat by the surgeon, and is slightly obstructed by the general swelling in the area.  What that means is that the urine now comes out not in a smooth, straight, stream but in more of a fan shape that changes position during urination and from day to day.  It can take up to three months for the swelling to go down enough for the urine stream to straighten out and become predictable, and until then the experience of peeing on various parts of your underside is something which you just have to get used to.  It's something which you also have to take extra time and effort to clean up afterwards in order to prevent infections.

The rest of the day was pretty much spent dilating, resting, talking, and eating.  Joan was scheduled to leave for the clinic soon after dinner, and it was during one of our afternoon dilation sessions that Anne and I heard a knock on our door.

"Who is it?" Anne asked.

"It's Joan", came the reply.

"We're dilating," Anne said.

I piped in and said, "Wait a minute, Joan."  Then I turned to Anne and said, "Maybe she needs to see this.  It can only help if she knows what she's going to be in for.  I don't have any objections to her coming in."

"Well, that's true," Anne replied, "And it wouldn't bother me to have her in here either."  Then she turned towards the door and called out, "Well, we're dilating, but you can come in if you want to."

We could see the top of the door open behind the folding screen that was set up between the doorway and the rest of the bedroom, then it closed again, and a moment later Joan stuck her head around the edge of the screen.  After a quick glance she stepped into the middle of the room and stood there for a few moments, silently glancing back at forth at the two of us who were naked from the waist down with our legs spread wide, our groin and upper thigh areas black and blue and swollen, and our white stents, slathered with KY jelly, sticking out of our vaginas. Finally, she took a deep breath and then slowly exhaled while pushed her extended hands (palms down) towards the floor as though trying to suppress something.  "OK," she muttered, "I can deal with this."  Then she sat down on the third bed and began asking us questions.

"Is the surgical site painful?"

"Much less now that the medical stents are out, but still quite sore.  Quick or large motions and sitting are very uncomfortable."

"Is dilating painful?"

"The #1 and #2 stents are not much problem.  The #3 stent is another thing, but we're hoping that will get easier as we do it more often.  It's still a little early to be sure."

"What does dilating feel like?"

"Physically, it's certainly a *different* experience, but there's really not much internal sensation at this point because the nerves are still pretty disoriented.  Maybe that will change in the future, but again, it's still too early to know.  Psychologically, it feels very strange, in an oddly fulfilling way.  It feels like this is the way we knew things always should have been, and it feels very comfortable, but at the same time it feels kind of strange that we should just be having this experience for the first time when we're in our 40's.  It's almost like our minds are wondering, 'Wait a minute ... what happened to those other decades?  Why hasn't this feeling been there for the past 40-plus years?  I just don't get it.'  Intellectually we know why, but emotionally it's kind of like having a sense that part of your past is missing and you're not quite sure what part that is or whether you should feel good or bad about it."

We all continued talking together for a while longer, with Anne and I also asking Joan how she was feeling about her impending surgery and trying to reassure her as best we could.  Finally, she left to begin packing her stuff for her trip to the clinic and to rest a bit before dinner.  Anne and I finished our session, cleaned up and douched, chatted a bit more, and then I think I took a nap while she went to the living room to visit with Lee and Barbara and watch a little TV.

At dinner time Joan was more quiet than usual and Lee, Barbara, Anne, and I spent extra time asking her how she was feeling and helping her "process" her thoughts and fears a bit.

Susan and Donna came back from the clinic for dinner and let us know that everything had gone well with Vicky and Beverly but that the two of them were still unconscious.  Susan and Donna were going back to the clinic for a short while after dinner, and the two of them and Barbara all offered to escort Joan over as well so that she would have some company and not feel alone. Lee and Anne and I were pleased when Joan accepted the offer. After Joan and the others had left, Anne and I went back upstairs for another round of dilations and, when that session was done, we both just went to sleep ... another night of rest interspersed with Moroccan-roll.

**Seven Days After Surgery:**

The first thing we got to do today (one week after surgery) was re-start taking our estrogen pills.  After three weeks of being off of them, it was a psychological "upper" to be able to include them in the daily routine again.  Most transsexuals (myself included, I must admit) have a psychological attachment to their hormone regimen which is just short of being an addiction. While the hormones are *not* magic potions and do *not*  produce quick, or easy, or inexpensive, or side-effect-free results, the fact remains that for many transsexuals (both male-to-female and female-to-male) they are what often produces the first really major physiological changes in our bodies and offer us (for the first time in our lives) a glimpse of the possibility of wholeness.  Having to stop taking them three weeks earlier, in preparation for surgery, had psychologically been rather difficult for me because of the internal fear that the "guy" me would somehow jump to the forefront again, against my will, once the female chemistry was reduced.  Now that surgery was over, and now that my little testosterone-producing factories had been permanently closed down, the importance of my psychological desire for estrogen had become secondary to the importance of taking them for medical reasons.  The human body apparently needs average levels of either estrogen or testosterone to help stave off certain degenerative diseases, such as osteoporosis.  Because of that, post-operative transsexuals (both FTM and MTF) need to continue with their hormone regimens for the rest of their lives in order to avoid some serious health problems.

After taking our pills, we began another day of dilations. It was only our second day dilating, but already the experience was getting old.  It seemed like all we were doing all day was lying on our backs inserting things into ourselves ... boring.  Well, maybe not boring, but certainly *not* intellectually stimulating. Mealtimes suddenly became a very interesting diversion.  After our first session we cleaned up and headed downstairs for breakfast, our chair survival kits in hand.  I had an incredible appetite!  Raphael, the chef, met us as we entered the dining area and, with his wonderful french accent, asked, "So, what would you two ladies like for breakfast this morning?"

I asked, "What have you got?"

With a big smile, he responded "*Anything* you want!"

"OK," I said, "I'll have toast, scrambled eggs, orange juice, and home fries."

His smile disappeared and without missing a beat, he shot back, "No home fries."

"Oh ........ well then, I'll have toast, scrambled eggs, and orange juice."  His smile returned.  "Excellent!" he exclaimed.

As we ate we all made note of the fact that Joan was probably in surgery and hoped among ourselves that everything was going well.  Donna and Susan joined us at the table for breakfast before they headed over to the clinic, and we asked them how Beverly and Vicky were doing.  Donna reported that Beverly seemed to be doing quite well and taking things in stride, but Susan told us that Vicky was having a very hard time with the pain, and she (Susan) seemed to be having quite a lot of emotional sympathy pain herself at seeing what her daughter was

going through.  We all did our best to comfort her, especially
Anne and I who had been through it ourselves, and she seemed
a bit heartened.

After a little more discussion Donna and Susan both
mentioned that they needed to get to a store to get some items
for themselves and their family members, and Barbara piped in
that she'd love to go to the stores as well, just to get out of the
house for a bit.  Anne and I looked at each other and then said
that we wanted to go too.  We each wanted to get some small
gifts for Vicky and Joan, and I needed to get some thigh-high
stockings to wear on my trip back to Maine.  Anne and I decided
to re-arrange our dilation schedule to fit in the shopping trip by
doing only one dilation between lunch and supper and adding an
extra dilation between supper and bedtime.  That meant that if
we all left right after lunch we would have about two hours available before we had to be back for the afternoon dilation.

After breakfast, Donna and Susan took off to spend the
morning at the clinic, Barbara and Lee returned to their room to
look after Lee's morning medical maintenance, and Anne and I
sat around for a while talking with staff members Raphael and
Annie before finally heading back to our room for dilation session
number two.

When that was over I read for a while and then took a
short nap before lunch.  Taking naps had become one of our fa-
vorite pastimes.  The surgery just seemed to sap all our strength,
and whatever alertness we were able to accumulate from an entire night of sleep seemed to disappear with very little exertion.  It
should not have surprised us, then, that our afternoon trip to the
stores would be so tiring, but as we piled into Donna's van after
lunch, that thought was furthest from our minds.

We went to the same little shopping mall that we'd all
been to before.  Mostly we just walked ... slowly ... taking small
steps ... and window shopped.  We had left our "donuts" and pillows in the van because we thought that carrying them around in

the mall might be too much of a distraction and that people would think it a bit too weird, but doing so meant that there was really no place we could sit if we got tired ... at least no place we could sit for more than 30 seconds or a minute, and then only by putting most of our weight on our tailbone rather than squarely on our butts.

I looked high and low for a place with items that inspired me to buy them, but nothing seemed quite right, and I was beginning to think that I would leave empty-handed when we came to a book/gift store and I noticed that it had a section of small, stained-glass, window hangings. I browsed through them and almost immediately found two that I knew would be perfect for Joan and Vicky. With those safely paid for and packed away, I was ready to leave. Anne was beginning to look a bit worn out as well. Donna, Susan, and Barbara wanted to go to another shopping center to continue their searches and little mini-vacations from the clinic, so it was decided that they would drop us off back at the residence and continue on. When Anne and I finally got back home we noted that we'd only been gone for an hour and a half. We were exhausted, and another nap was called for before we could begin our third dilation session.

Maybe is was just the combination of being physically tired, intellectually bored, and spiritually energized, but our third dilation, just before dinner, was completely wacky. I think it started when Anne made some kind of risque remark and I, very straight-faced, shot back a response that sent her into a fit of laughter. Once it got started it just seemed to build on itself as we each tried to come up with funnier and funnier comebacks. In a few minutes we were laughing so hard we were crying and found that we were having a hard time keeping the stents in place because laughing would compress the stomach and groin muscles and pop the stents out, like little missiles, almost as fast as we could reinsert them. We also found that compressing those stomach and groin muscles was actually somewhat painful, but there seemed to be nothing we could do to stop.

Because of that, we were a little relieved when Dr. Brassard came into the room to check up on how we were doing.  It gave us someone else to focus on.  Almost simultaneously Anne and I each reached for the remaining dilator in its anti-bacterial bath and, holding them like aspergillums, began sprinkling him as though with holy water.

He smiled widely and chuckled and then asked us how the dilations were going.  We quickly filled him in on our experiences (especially the pain we were having with the #3 dilator) and asked a few questions about the techniques we were using and what we should be expecting in the line of changes over the next days and weeks.  We also continued to shoot jokes back-and-forth.  He listened with a smile on his face, answered our questions, and, when we could think of nothing else to ask him, excused himself and left.  Almost immediately Anne and I were back into hysterical laughter, the silliness continuing through the rest of the session.

When we were through, we began (amid continuing chuckles) to gather up our dilators, and towels, and douches, and paper towels, and clothes, and brushes, and whatever before heading for the bathroom.  Anne had her hands full and a hair scrungie in her mouth, and when I asked her if she had everything she said (through clenched teeth), "I need a tchow."

I asked, "A what?"

She responded, more emphatically, "A TCHOW!"

"A cow!" I exclaimed ... "Why do you want a cow?"

Her mouth opened wide in laughter, the scrungie fell to the floor, and she screamed, "Stop it!  Stop it ... it hurts!!"  She was right, the harder we laughed, the more it hurt, but the more we looked at each other, the harder we laughed.  With our arms full of supplies, we staggered from the bedroom, entered the second-level hallway (which overlooked the living room), and headed for the bathroom.  As we slowly made our way down the hall, partly doubled over from laughter and pain, I glanced down into the living room and saw Lee, Barbara, and Marie-Andree following us silently with their eyes.  On their faces were the unmistakable half-grins of wonder that people get when they observe someone who they are sure is crazy.

It turned out that they weren't the only ones who were amused.  Later, when we went down to dinner, Lee asked, "What were you guys doin' up there?!  We heard you laughin' all the way in the living room!  When Dr. Brassard came down, he sat at the kitchen table and fell apart laughin'!  He said, 'They're sprinkling like priests!'  What's that all about!?"  We did our best to explain it all, but I'm afraid it just wasn't as funny the second time around.

After dinner we still had two dilations to do.  The first of them went fairly well, though the #3 dilator continued to be painful and actually seemed to be getting worse as the vagina continued to try closing up, the muscles slowly continued to "wake up" from the shock of surgery, and the nerves in the crotch area continued to heal and once again send out their little pain messages.

With the fourth dilation session done, we went down to the living room to rest and chat for a while with whoever else was around.  Sylvia, stopped by for a few minutes and we expressed our concern about the problems we heard Vicky was having with her pain.  She replied that it was not uncommon for younger clients to have trouble handling the pain of surgery, something which she ascribed to the fact that they generally were less emotionally mature and tended to have had fewer experiences in life in dealing with physical adversity.  Nevertheless, she reassured us that the nurses and doctors were doing everything they could to help ease Vicky's experience.

After what seemed like a very short time in the living room, we trudged back upstairs (at about 8:30 p.m.) to start the

final dilation session of the day.  The combination of the late-
ness, our tiredness from the afternoon excursion, our being worn
out from the afternoon laugh fest, and our general weakness
made this final dilation a more tiring and painful one than usual.
Anne and I both  experienced a lot of pain from the #3 dilator.
Anne's pain was so severe that she could not hold the dilator in
for more than a few minutes and had to replace it with the #2
dilator to finish the session.  A little later, when we had finished
up and were lying in our beds waiting to fall into sleep, we talked
about the situation and decided to alter the dilation schedule in
an attempt to get around the pain by exposing ourselves to it for
less time.  The next morning we would go from the 3-5-25 minute
schedule and instead do a 5-7-21 minute schedule (5 minutes
with #1, 7 minutes with #2, and 21 minutes with #3).  It would be
an experiment, but we felt that we had to do something, and with
the decision made I fell into another night of two-hour blocks of
sleep and Moroccan-roll.

**Eight Days After Surgery:**

The days now seem to be rushing by and are pretty
much an undifferentiated blur of dilations, naps, eating, and chatting.  In two more days we will be leaving our new home to return
to families and friends and (eventually) jobs and the rest of our
lives.  It feels like I just got here yesterday!

The first and second dilations, if anything, seem even a
little more painful with the #3 dilator, and we are now approaching each session with gritted teeth and a sense of dread.  The #1
and #2 dilators are fine, and the #3 dilator is *only* 1/8 inch larger
in diameter than #2, but that 1/8 inch seems to make all the difference and sends the muscles around the new vaginal opening
into a real tizzy.  The inner thigh muscles are also affected because they criss-cross and connect onto the pelvis in the same

area so that not only our crotch is in pain but our whole upper-inner-thigh.

After the second session Anne decided unilaterally to once again rearrange her dilation schedule to give her more time with the #2 dilator, going from a 5-7-21 minute schedule to a 5-14-14 minute schedule. I decided to stay on the old schedule.

We had the opportunity to go shopping again but turned it down so that we could rest more, get dressed a bit, and go visit Beverly, Vicky, and Joan in the clinic. After lunch we did another painful dilation session, got dressed, and headed for the clinic on foot. It was a beautiful fall day out, the air was fresh and brisk, and the 15-minute walk actually felt good to our leg muscles which were a bit cramped from the tension they always seemed to be under.

At the clinic we found Donna and Beverly chatting and watching television in Beverly's room. Beverly certainly did seem to be doing well with the whole experience. She was alert, talkative, and claimed that she really didn't find the pain to be too bad at all. Having been through it, I couldn't imagine it myself, and personally felt that I detected a bit of pretense, but I said nothing about it and expressed my happiness at finding her do-ing so well.

In Vicky and Joan's room the situation was a little differ-ent. Vicky made no bones about the pain she was experiencing or how she felt about it, and she made sure to ask us how long we thought it would last and what she could do about it once she was back at the residence. We tried to reassure her that the first couple of days after surgery were the hardest (and they were) and that she would soon be up and walking around, which would be very helpful in lessening her discomfort. We also offered some thoughts on how to avoid/handle her pain once she was back at the residence.

Joan, who had just had her surgery the day before, was still pretty much out of things, and we found her in deep sleep ...

or maybe it was morphine-unconsciousness.  We gave Vicky her gifts, which she thought were very sweet, and left Joan's by her bed where she would eventually discover them once she was alert enough.  Then, we left and headed back to the residence.

The whole visit had lasted maybe 15 minutes, and the total time for the trip to the clinic and back home again was less than an hour, but it still managed to wear us out.  After getting back into our pajamas we both settled in for yet another nap.

During the fourth dilation session, just before supper, Anne had *BIG* trouble with the #3 dilator.  The pain she was feeling was so bad that she began to cry and I urged her to remove the #3 stent and finish the session with the #2 ... a suggestion that she was more than willing to take.  Unfortunately, during the time that she had the #3 stent in place the pain had moved to her upper thighs and the muscles had cramped so that when we were finished she was still experiencing a lot of discomfort.  As soon as I could get up, I went over to her bed and went to work massaging her legs as she bit her lips and cried a little more.  Then I held her for a while to comfort her as she muttered things like, "Oh, God, that was awful" and "I don't want to do that again."

The pain that *I* had been feeling with the #3 dilator was borderline bearable, and I should have taken Anne's reaction as a warning, but being the stoic and stubborn person that I am I had pushed it out of my mind and concentrated on helping Anne deal with her pain.  It was a big mistake.  During the fifth, and last, session of the day I found out just how big a mistake it was.

Both of us dreaded that final session, but Sylvia's in-structions had seemed pretty emphatic that using the #3 dilator was necessary if we wanted to maintain what we had spent dec-ades of our lives working to achieve, so we both began with the determination to do what we needed to do.

The #1 and #2 dilators, as usual, were no problem. When it came time for the #3 dilator we both kind of silently shook our heads, clenched our teeth, and slowly pushed it into place.  Anne lasted about five minutes and then exclaimed, "I can't take it any more ... I'm going back to #2!", and I wordlessly nodded my acknowledgement.  In my stupidity I was determined to keep mine in for the whole 21 minutes, though my jaw was now firmly clenched from the physical tension that was building in my body.  I put on my earphones, found a radio station with some english-language music on it, cranked the volume up high, closed my eyes, and focused all my attention onto the words and the music, blocking out the pain messages from my body.

When the session time was over I turned off the radio, took a deep breath, and reached for the dilator to remove it, only to find that the vaginal and thigh muscles were now so tense and contracted that the damn thing didn't want to come out!  At this point my attention was just about completely on the pain I was feeling, and after twisting the dilator back and forth a little to get it loosened up I was finally able to slowly extract it from myself.  As the tip of the dilator was finally withdrawn and the vaginal muscles, now free to contract, clamped the opening closed, all hell broke loose.  Two huge bolts of pain shot down my legs, sending them into convulsions, and a similar bolt felt like it was ricochetting around inside my torso, jerking me repeatedly into a semi-fetal position.  My breath was coming in gasps, and I was crying freely.  Anne came rushing over from her bed and tried to massage my legs, but I was moving around so much that she decided instead to sit on the bed and just hold me until things subsided a bit.  In a minute or so, when the convulsions had pretty much gone and the gasping had turned into heavy breathing, she was finally able to get to work on my leg muscles and massaged them for several minutes while they continued to twitch and I continued to cry.

As the muscles relaxed, as the pain lessened, as my breathing became easier and slower, and as more clarity returned to my brain, I began to feel more and more stupid.  Finally, I looked up at Anne, flashed a big grin, and said, "I don't think I'll do that again."

She grinned back at me, gave her head a little shake, and said, "Honey, you had me worried!  Don't do that again."

After we had finished cleaning up we returned to our room for a few minutes and reclined on our beds, talking, trying to figure out what to do about the #3 dilator.  Maintaining depth in the vagina wasn't a concern as all three dilators were the same length and we could maintain depth with the #1 and #2 dilators.  It was the diameter that was bothering us, combined with the post-surgical sensitivity of the muscles and nerves.  I wanted to rearrange the dilation schedule to eliminate the #3 dilator completely, at least for a while, until more healing had taken place and the muscles in the area were more comfortable with their new state-of-being. "Besides," I argued, pulling the #3 dilator out of its bath and holding it up in front of us, "Ain't nobody that big *ever* comin' near me!"

"Well of course not," Anne replied, "you're lesbian.  But I'm not!"

"Look," I asked, "how many guys have you met who are that big?"

She glanced at the stent. "Not many."

"And have you felt sexually attracted to any of them?"

"No."

"OK.  So let's assume a worst-case scenario.  Suppose you're right and we stop using the #3 stent for a while and then find that we can't go back to using it later on.  That means that you might not be able to comfortably handle anyone larger than the #2 stent.  But for heaven's sake, with *that* you can still handle maybe 99% of the men that you might find yourself attracted to! Why would you want to hurt yourself for a 1% who you'll probably never even run into?"

I was making headway, and Anne was mostly agreeable, but she still felt that stopping the #3 dilator completely might make it too difficult to re-start using it later.  In the end we decided to rearrange the dilations to an 8-20-4 minute schedule, giving most of the time to the #2 dilator and, we hoped, enough time to the #3 dilator while keeping our pain to a minimum.  With that decision made we both went down to the living room to chat for a while with whoever we could find and perhaps get some milk and cookies.

At about 9:00 p.m. I decided to turn in and left Anne and the other folks in the living room.  Back in the bedroom, I closed the curtains and lay in bed, the light still on, thinking about the past two weeks and the whole lifetime that had led up to them.  Anne came in about an hour later and, seeing that I was still awake, chatted quietly with me for a while, joining me in reviewing and analyzing our experiences.

At last we both decided it was time to sleep, and Anne turned off the light on her headboard, leaving the room illuminated by the little bit of light that filtered in from the street.  In the quiet and the darkness I felt very calm and centered, my mind almost empty of thoughts; but somewhere deep down inside me, in the area of my solar plexus, I could feel an uneasiness of some kind vibrating and growing.  Then suddenly, like a floodgate opening, I began to cry ... long, heartfelt, sobs that just seemed to come out of nowhere.  Anne turned on her bed-light again and looked over at me.

"What's wrong?"

"I don't know," I answered between tears.

"Are you in pain?"

"No," I responded in a little wail.

Anne got out of bed and came over to me.  I rose into a sitting position and she sat on the edge of my bed, putting her arms around me.  My sobs came faster and heavier.

"What's the problem?" she asked quietly.

"I honestly don't know.  I don't know where this is coming from."

She held me for some minutes as I continued to cry.  I really *didn't* know where the tears were coming from.  I didn't feel sad, at least not any kind of feeling that I could identify as sad.  Still, there *was* a feeling of some kind there, a feeling that I couldn't put my finger on, something that I couldn't remember ever having felt before, but which felt very primal.

Suddenly there was a light knock on our bedroom door and staff member Marie-Andree, herself a post-op, came in with a concerned look on her face.  She had heard me crying from down in the living room.

"Is something wrong?" she asked.

"No, not really," Anne replied.  "She's just having a bit of emotional release."

Marie-Andree left, and I continued to cry as Anne held me, but about a minute later the door opened again and Marie-Andree came back in.  Without saying a word she came over to the other side of my bed, sat down, and simply took one of my hands in hers and held it.  I cried for some minutes more and then, feeling physically drained, though still in emotional turmoil, I lay back on my pillow with Anne and Marie-Andree sitting on either side of me, holding my hands.  My mind was racing.  The feeling that I couldn't put my finger on was very slowly coming together in my brain but still wasn't quite concrete enough to verbalize.

"How are you feeling?" Marie-Andree asked.

"Just very weak," I answered.  I laid quietly for a few moments with my eyes closed and then, looking up at both of them, I asked, "Why did we have to do that?  Why did we have to go through all of this *shit* that we've gone through just to be who we are?"  And as the words came out, the feeling came into focus, and I realized what it was ...... I was feeling anger.  I was angry about the nearly four decades of my life that were gone and which I could never get back, the four decades when I worked so hard to hide who I was so that other people could feel comfortable with me.  I was angry about the decades of guilt that I'd had to live with in order to be acceptable to the world, the decades of loneliness as I kept my inner self away from everyone else so that they wouldn't find out about me, the decades of fear that being found out would mean hatred or rejection from my friends and family, the decades of emotional pain that came from feeling like some kind of freak.

Where I was now was better ... it was so, SO much better, and felt so much more comfortable and natural, simply being me, simply being who I was.  But, God, what a price I had had to pay, what a price we had all had to pay, to get there:  all those years, all that loneliness, all that emotional turmoil, all that physical pain, and (for some of us) all that hatred, rejection, and discrimination thrown in our faces.  What right did the world have to do that to us?  I was angry that it did.  I was angry that I fell for it. I was angry because, for the first time in my life, I could let that anger out without having to worry about the consequences.  I was *ME*, finally, and if the world didn't like it there was nothing it could do to change it or keep it from me.

My questions to Anne and Marie-Andree had been short and simple, but they intuitively knew exactly what I meant and where I was coming from.  Anne looked down at me, gave my hand a squeeze, and said simply, "We don't have to worry about it any more.  We're home now."

Marie-Andree smiled a little and said, "You know, a year from now this will all seem like a dream.  You'll look back on it and wonder,  'Did I really go through all of that?'  You'll look back at that other person that you were before and you won't even be able to remember being that way ... it will just feel like you've always been the way you are now.  Trust me, I know ... all the pain will go away."

Anne got up without saying a word and left the room, to go to the bathroom I supposed.  Marie-Andree smiled and said,

"You know, it's been good for me to sit and talk with you a little.
It's helped to ease my headache."

"You have a headache?" I asked, and without saying
another word I reached up and began massaging her forehead
and temples.  She closed her eyes and said nothing while I gently massaged her for several minutes more.  When I finally
stopped she opened her eyes, smiled down at me, and then
leaned over and gave me a big, silent hug.  Straightening up,
she asked, "Are you going to be OK now?"

"Yes, I think so," I replied with a smile as she got up to
leave.

Anne came back into the room just as Marie-Andree was
leaving and, after talking with me for another minute or so to
make sure I was OK, climbed back into her bed and turned off
the light.  That night I slept very well ... no Moroccan-roll.

## Nine Days After Surgery:

This was our last day at the residence.  Tomorrow we
would both leave to go home and in some ways we were already
feeling homesick for the residence, the place where we had our
new births.  The day itself was pretty unremarkable, just more of
the same: dilating, eating, napping, and chatting; but the chat
seemed more low-key, and our voices were just a little tinged
with sadness over our impending separation from the place and
from each other.

We were now on the re-arranged 8-20-4 minute dilation
schedule that we decided on the night before.  Even just four
minutes with the #3 dilator felt like a long, very painful time.  Still,
it was just shy of being unbearable, so we continued with it
throughout the day.

Dr. Menard arrived at the residence in the afternoon, and
the three of us went up to our bedroom for a final inspection and
some medical treatment.

I remember thinking that, while everything seemed per-
fectly natural to the three of us, it would probably have been a
slightly comical scene to anyone who was unfamiliar with the
circumstances and who happened in on it.  Anne and I were in
our bathrobes, once again naked from the waist down (seems
like we did a lot of that), lying on our beds, propped up on our
elbows, legs spread, listening intently to this man (with his
French accent and impeccable three-piece suit) as he stood between us with a flashlight in one hand and a pair of surgical scissors in the other, instructing us on proper medical care and hygiene.

When he had gone over all the information he needed to
tell us he went to work removing two or three small stitches that
had been purposely left in place for more than a week.  These
stitches were holding a small flap of skin over the new clitoris,
giving it some added protection while it started healing.  Once
the neo-clitoris was freed, his next-to-the-last task was taking
some photos of the surgical site which he could use later to
check on his work and to compare (when we came back for our
6-month check-up) against how things actually ended up healing.
He asked if it would be all right with us for him to take the photos,
emphasizing that they would only be photos of his surgery, not
our faces, and we both readily agreed.

His camera was a 35mm SLR with a special close-up
lens that had a light built into its rim ... very fancy ... and I could
tell he enjoyed playing it.  Anne went first, and as he approached
her I cried out in mock horror, "Don't do it, Anne!  What if you
want to run for public office?!"  He glanced at me with a grin on
his face and chuckled loudly.

When all of that was done, he returned to the middle of
the room at the foot of our beds, told us that we had been "good"
patients and that he and the staff had enjoyed having us there,
and then asked if we had any final questions.  As it happened,
Anne and I had been writing down questions for him as we had

been thinking of them over the previous two or three days so, yes, we *did* have questions ... a whole page of them. I will summarize them here for those of you who might be interested in knowing what was on our minds and how Dr. Menard answered.

Q: For how long will the #3 dilator cause us pain?
A: Until the area is pretty much healed and the muscles in the area are more flexible and used to their new condition.

Q: When can we expect the swelling in the pubic area to diminish?
A: It usually begins to diminish about 2-3 weeks after surgery and takes another 2-3 weeks to complete.

Q: When can we expect to be able to urinate normally?
A: Generally, when the swelling in the area goes down, but it may take as long as three months.

Q: Aside from the normal, daily hygiene routine, can we expect anything else to cause pain problems?
A: Not really, only an infection if you are not careful about keeping the area clean and the suture lines covered with anti-biotic cream. For the next 2-3 weeks, the more soaking baths (using anti-bacterial soap) that you can take, the greater and faster will be your healing.

Q: We understand that at home we should be dilating four times a day for the next 1 1/2 to 2 months and then go down to three times a day for a while and eventually (after about six months) be at a couple of times a week. Is that sufficient?
A: Everyone is different. You have the dilation schedule that we gave you to take home with you. If you follow that everything should be fine, but that is basically just a guideline. The real idea is that at first you need to be dilating four times per day until

doing so becomes very easy and painless and the dilators go in without any trouble or discomfort (should take 1 1/2 to 2 months). When you reach that point, then you go to three dilations per day and stay there for another 1 1/2 to 2 months....then you go to two dilations per day for a few months, then one dilation a day for a few months, and so on until you get it down to once or twice a week.

Q:  Any special medical tests or issues that we need to be relaying to our doctors and keeping an eye on in the future?
A:  You need now to be just as careful about urinary tract infections as any woman would be.  You should be having a yearly PAP smear and visual exam of the walls of the new vagina just as any other woman should be getting.

Q:  Continued prostate exams?  How should those be done?
A:  You still have your prostates, but because of the lack of testosterone and the presence of estrogen in your systems they have probably gotten *very* small and may even be difficult to locate by palpation.  It certainly wouldn't hurt to check it every now and then, but now you have a vagina located between the colon and the prostate, so if your doctor wants to palpate the prostate it would better be done through the vagina because that is closer.

Q:  How much leeway do we have in altering the depth and width of the vagina with dilation?  Suppose we wanted to *not* use the #3 dilator for a while but wanted to go back to using it later on, would we lose that ability?
A:  The depth of the new vagina can be maintained with any of the dilators because they are all the same length.  The vagina I've made for you is about five inches deep, but by putting just a little bit of extra pressure on the dilator while you dilate you may be able to stretch it over several months to get an additional 1/2 inch or one inch, but probably not more.  The diameter of the

new vagina will depend on which is the largest diameter stent that you end up dilating with.  If you want to not use the largest stent for a little while, that will not cause any irreversible setbacks as long as you go back to using it eventually.  But you cannot wait for too long a time.  Generally speaking, you have roughly a year (the time it takes for complete healing to occur) to make changes in the depth and width of the vagina, after that it is pretty much set and you would have a hard time changing it.

Q:  How long should dead skin be sloughing off from the inside of the vagina?
A:  Certainly for the next three to four weeks, but it could take as long as two to three months.

Q:  Can we do too much douching?
A:  No.

Q:  Can we do too little douching?
A:  Well, if you don't douche at all, that would be too little douching.  For the next few months or so, while things are still healing, sutures are still coming out, and dead skin is still sloughing off it would be good to douche at least twice a day, morning and evening.  After that you can slowly lessen the frequency until you are douching maybe once or twice a week, if you want to do it that infrequently.

Q:  Is there anything we can do to make dilations easier, or will that only come with time?
A:  That will only come with time.

Q:  When can we get back to physical exercise and how strenuous should it be?

A:  You should be able to start exercising again in a couple of weeks, but one month would be better.  Just start off light and slowly work your way up.  Don't cause yourself pain or fatigue.

    With all of that done he bid us good-bye for the evening, saying that he might be around in the morning before we left. We thanked him for his work and said that we hoped to see him again, and then he was gone.
    Anne and I chatted a bit more, going over our notes and making sure that we both understood all the things he had told us, and by then it was time for our pre-dinner dilation.
    When it was over and we had cleaned up, we went downstairs for dinner where I discovered that my friend who was driving me back to Maine (Michelle...an MTF pre-op) had already arrived and made herself at home with everyone.  I knew she was coming but, in a way, it was actually strange and jarring to see her.  For two weeks I'd really not had any contact, other than a few phone calls, with any of my Maine friends and family.  All of my focus, attention, and being had been invested in the clinic and the residence, and it was almost as though Maine had ceased to exist.  All that existed was this new life I had entered. Now, suddenly, here was Maine and the life I had left behind (all in the form of poor, unsuspecting, Michelle) standing in front of me and waiting to take me back, and I didn't want *anything* to do with it!!
    Luckily, I realized why I was feeling so negatively emo-tional about seeing her and as soon as I could I took her aside and said, "Michelle, I don't want you to feel like I'm ignoring you or anything, but these last few weeks have really been an in-credible emotional experience, and the experience is still going on and I'm still processing it, so if I seem a little withdrawn and don't pay too much attention to you, please bear with me and don't take it personally, OK?"  She was totally cool with that,

thank heavens, and readily agreed to leave me alone while I re-focused myself.

Dinner was a little more energized than usual, what with Michelle joining us as well as two new pre-ops who would be having their surgery the following Monday.  Three new faces in the crowd meant a whole new slew of ideas and subjects to talk about as well as another round of questions aimed at Lee and Anne and me about what our experience had been like.  It helped give my mind a little diversion from the realization that it was all about to end.  Still, every now and then I found myself glancing over at Michelle (and the "other" life that she repre-sented) as a way to remind myself of what was coming and slowly get myself used to the idea.  I guess it worked, because by the time Anne and I went up to our room for the evening dila-tion I was feeling comfortable enough to have Michelle join us, and the three of us chatted away like high-school girls at an ice-cream parlor until it was time to go to sleep.

I didn't sleep very well that night.  I tossed and turned and seemed to spend more time with my eyes open rather than closed; but eventually I dozed off and didn't wake until about 6:00 am.

# RECUPERATION AT HOME

**Ten Days After Surgery:**

This turned out to be a short day at the residence and a long day on the road, which is exactly what I was expecting it to be.

Anne and I got up early and did our pre-breakfast dilation, followed by some packing. Anne had a plane to catch to get back home, so we had a quick breakfast with everyone, after which we all gathered in the living room for the taking of the traditional photos of the post-ops (photos which are then placed in a big photo album for subsequent clients to look through ... kind of like a high school year book). Dr. Menard came by for a few minutes and we both got to thank him again for his fine work.

After that, Anne and I went back up to our room and finished packing, working quickly but talking the whole time. Then her ride to the airport came, we hugged, said good-bye, promised to keep in touch, and before I knew it she was gone and I was suddenly feeling like a rudderless ship, drifting without direction.

Now I didn't have a choice ... now I *had* to refocus on my Maine life and my support system of friends and family ... now I *had* to relegate the past two weeks to my memory and my heart and once again take up the banalities of making a living and living a life. It was a big emotional let-down.

Michelle helped me load my stuff into her car and, after spending a few more minutes sharing good-bye's and hugs with Lee and Barbara and Raphael and Marie-Andree and whoever else was there that morning, we got in and drove off, heading for the clinic.  It was actually right on the route as we headed out of town, and I wanted to say good-bye to the folks who were there as well.  This was the day that they would all be returning to the residence.

Beverly and Donna were both chipper and wished me well.  Vicky actually seemed to be doing a little better and talked much less about any pain she was feeling.  Her biggest interest seemed to be in the dilation process and exactly how it was done.  I told her not to worry about it, that the folks at the residence would do a very good job in explaining and teaching it to her, and I quickly dispelled her impression that it was done by moving the dilator repeatedly in and out. "No," I said, "it just goes in and you hold it in for however many minutes it's supposed to be there.  You don't move it back and forth."

Joan was awake during this visit.  She thanked me for the gift I had left her, said that she *was* in some pain but that she would be able to put up with it, and asked how my experience had been at the residence over the past three days.  We talked a bit longer, and then I said good-bye and went back out to the car.

As we were driving off, I turned to Michelle, explained that I really wasn't feeling very talkative at the moment, and asked her not to be upset if I just sat quietly for a while.  "You talk when you're ready," she replied.

The ride home was really uneventful.  I was already feeling tired from the little bit of exertion that I had done that morning, so I put the seat back, stuffed a pillow behind my head, and did my best to sleep, falling in and out of consciousness.  When I was awake I would think to myself about the previous two weeks.  After about an hour I put the seat up a bit and just quietly looked out the window.  Every now and then, feeling guilty about the silence I was subjecting Michelle to, I would make small talk for a few moments.  I nodded in and out of sleep.  My crotch felt *very* sore, but it was not unbearable, and I made every effort to simply not move since that seemed to be the plan that worked best.

In about two hours we were back in the States, and in another hour I asked Michelle to pull over at an information center and rest stop in Vermont so that I could go to the bathroom.

I still had to be very careful about infections and, since I was actually dressed (not in the night-gown and slippers that I had practically lived in for the past two weeks), this little rest stop turned into quite a production number.

First I had to pick a stall to go into, and I opted for the handicapped stall because it was so spacious and I had plenty of room to move around in.

Next, I had to clean the toilet as best I could and I made several trips between the bathroom sink and the toilet with wet and then dry paper towels.

After that I doused several paper towels with as much water as they would hold and took those and several other dry towels into the stall with me, hanging them on the handicapped grab bars around the toilet.

Then I stripped from the waist down, slowly taking each of my thigh-high stockings off and immediately putting my foot back into my shoe so that I wouldn't have to put my bare feet on the cold, dingy tile floor.

At that point I was ready to urinate and, after all the preparation it had taken, I savored every moment.

Personal cleanup consisted of a first pass with toilet paper, followed by the wet paper towels (since no bidet was available), followed by the dry paper towels, followed by a last pass with toilet paper.  Toilet paper went into the toilet, paper towels went temporarily onto the floor until I was finished.  Then I got out my little mirror and my tube of anti-biotic cream and re-anointed all the suture lines.  After that a fresh panty liner went into my underwear and I got re-dressed.  I repacked all my stuff, cleaned up the stall a bit (throwing the paper towels and old panty liner into the garbage can), washed my hands, and headed back out to the car, a mere 20 minutes after I had entered.

An hour an a half later we stopped again, in New Hampshire, to get some lunch.  I was in the mood for an actual get-out-of-the-cramped-car-and-sit-in-a-nice-restaurant meal, so we passed up on McDonald's, Burger King, and the other fast-food places and went into a little family-style restaurant on the main street.  In any other situation I might have thought for a second before walking into such a place carrying a pillow and a cushion to sit on, but there was really no choice since I simply couldn't sit without using them.  After slowly lowering myself onto the chair survival kit (several times), I was finally able to get into a position that was bearable and Michelle and I ended up having a very pleasant lunch and close conversation.

About another hour and a half after getting back on the road we stopped again so that I could once more use the bathroom, and the production number from the morning was repeated so as to avoid infection.

At this point I was well on my way to getting a major headache, caused by strained neck muscles from trying to sleep in the moving car.  I knew from personal experience that once I had reached that point there was no way to get rid of the neck pain (and the associated throbbing behind my eyeball) except to get into a real bed and sleep it off.

We finally reached my friend Marty's house, where I would be staying for the next five weeks; and even though the soreness in my crotch had not gotten any worse, the seven hours on the road had completely exhausted me and my neck-and-head ache was in full swing.  I did my best to greet Marty cheerfully and talk with her a bit about the ride back, but I really wasn't in the mood for anything except getting into bed.  Within about half an hour I had unpacked as much stuff as I would need immediately and I settled in to do my second (and last) dilation for the day.  The #3 dilator was particularly painful that evening, but I still managed to keep it in for the four minutes that Anne and I had decided on.  As I lay there with my stents, my head throbbing and my eyes closed, I could hear Marty and Michelle talking in the kitchen.  Marty was asking Michelle how she thought I was doing and how painful she thought the trip back might have been for me.

With the dilation session out of the way, I cleaned up, called down to Marty and Michelle to let them know I was going to sleep, crawled into bed, and slowly drifted off into dream-land. I missed my Moroccan-roll.

**Eleven Days After Surgery - Until I Start Work Again (Seven Weeks):**

This whole seven-week period is really easy to tell you about because (except for small changes or infrequent, noteworthy events) it was pretty much seven weeks of exactly the same, boring schedule, day in and day out.

This is what the whole daily schedule consisted of:

***   Wake up at about 6:00 am, go into the bathroom, brush my teeth, put my hair up out of the way, and take a five minute soaking bath.

***   Return to my room, make the bed and set it up for the day's first dilation session.

***   Dilate. (session #1)

***   Clean up afterwards, which sometimes meant a complete shower and washing my hair, but which usually involved washing only from the waist down (using the hand-held, flexible shower-head that Marty had in her shower).

***   At about 8:00 a.m. to 8:30 a.m., go downstairs and make something for breakfast.

***   From about 9:00 a.m. until 10:30 a.m., free time to chat, do emailing, rest, read, make fairly ineffectual plans for the day, etc.

***   At 10:30 am, go back upstairs and undress, prep the bed for dilation session #2, and take a five minute soaking bath.

***   Dilate. (session #2)

***   Clean up afterwards, including washing from the waist down.

***   Get dressed and, at about 12:00 noon, go downstairs for lunch.

***   From about 12:30 p.m. until about 3:30 p.m., free time to chat, do emailing, take a nap (which happened often), read, take a 15-minute walk around the neighborhood, or go into town with Marty to buy groceries or whatever.

***   At 3:30 p.m., go back upstairs and undress, prep the bed for dilation session #3, and take a five minute soaking bath.

***   Dilate. (session #3)

***   Clean up afterwards, including washing from the waist down.

***   Either get dressed again or stay in my pajamas and, about 5:00 p.m., go downstairs for supper.

***   From about 6:00 p.m. until 7:30 p.m., free time to chat, email, read, maybe watch a movie.

***   At 7:30 p.m., go back upstairs and undress, prep the bed for dilation session #4, and take a five minute soaking bath.

***   Dilate. (session #4)

***   Clean up afterwards, including washing from the waist down.

***   Put on my pajamas and, about 8:30 p.m., go downstairs for a snack and a chat.

***   At about 9:00 p.m., go to bed.

As you can imagine, that schedule quickly began to bore me.  I am, after all, a pretty active person and am always feeling the need to be doing something.  Nevertheless, I realized that this was really a once-in-a-lifetime situation, and that the things I did during this month-and-a-half would affect how well and how quickly I healed, which in turn would effect not only how soon I could get back into real activity but also how much and what kind of activity I would be able to engage in for the rest of my life. Having gotten this far, I didn't want to ruin my chances for a quick and complete recovery, so I kept a low profile and made myself stick with being fairly inactive and bored for the next six weeks.  I'm glad I did.

Physically, my energy level during this whole time was very low.  I tired easily, napped frequently, and about once a week seemed to hit a physiological block of some kind that forced me into bed where I would usually sleep for 12 or 14 hours straight.  My pain level was really not too bad, but the pain I had was continuously present and its consistency alone became a trial.  Nevertheless, it slowly receded over the days and weeks.  Sitting was always a problem, and I was usually walking around with a couple pillows and a cushion.  Marty kept an eye on me and soon figured out which arrangement of pillows and cushions I would use for any given chair, often having them prearranged for me when I would arrive in the kitchen to eat or head for the computer to do some emailing.  Early on, my upper thigh muscles began to cramp badly because I was unconsciously trying to shift my body weight (while sitting) from my butt to my legs ... kind of like the effect you might get if you went into a squat and tried to hold the position for half an hour or so.  Massages were somewhat helpful for getting rid of that discomfort, but ultimately I simply had to be mindful of what I was doing while sitting and put up with the crotch discomfort for a while in order to avoid the leg cramps for a longer period.

For the most part, dilations went very smoothly.  However, the #3 dilator, even at four minutes per session, was just too painful to take, and within a few days of arriving at Marty's place I had opted to stop using it completely for a while, going to a schedule of 10 minutes with the #1 dilator and 25 minutes with the #2 dilator.  I emailed Anne about what I had done and she responded that she was also still having lots of trouble with the #3 stent and had pretty much decided to stop using it as well (my decision being the impetus to carry through on the idea).  So, for the next seven weeks my dilations were done with just the #1 and #2 dilators.

Because urinating during the first month or so was such a process, what with all the cleaning up and washing afterwards in order to avoid infections, I finally opted (strange as it may seem) to simply stand up in the bathtub to pee and then wash myself and the tub down with the shower head when I was through.  Since I was usually just wearing my underwear with a bathrobe over it, the process was not as involved as it at first sounds.  However, like many good ideas, this one was quick to go bad.  I was already washing myself from the waist down before and after each dilation session (for a total of eight times a day).  With an added four times a day urinating, and usually another visit to the bathroom at some point during the night, I was ending up washing and drying my bottom half at least a dozen times every 24 hours.  That, coupled with the fact that Marty's house has VERY hard water, meant that it took less than a week for all of the skin on my legs, butt, and feet to become very, very dry and chapped.  Crevasses that were very painful started to show up on my soles and ankles, my knees became like sandpaper, and my thighs and calves broke out into an incredibly itchy rash.  I tried using body lotion after each washing in order to keep the skin moisturized, but it didn't help.  What I needed was to cut down on the number of times I was washing.  Thankfully, Marty suggested that I use a perry bottle (a little, plastic, spray bottle) and loaned me one that she had among her nursing things.  With it I was able to squat over the toilet and wash just those areas around the vagina and rectum that needed to be washed, allowing the rest of my lower body to replenish the natural body oils that I had been so assiduously removing.  Now I was down to just four baths a day, one before each dilation session, and in about a week the rash and chapping had pretty much disappeared.

About a week after I arrived at Marty's house she came in to talk with me for a bit during one of my dilation sessions. As she was leaving, she turned around and asked, "Do you always dilate lying on your back like that?"  I told her I did, and she asked, "You don't find it difficult?"  When I told her that I didn't find it difficult at all, just very boring because there wasn't much I could do while lying on my back, she said, "Well, why don't you sit up while you're dilating?"

"You mean like in a chair?  Can I do that?"

"No, not in a chair, but you can prop some pillows up behind you so you're maybe at a 45 degree angle.  That would make it easier to reach where you have to go and give you the ability to at least hold a book or something so you wouldn't have to be staring at the ceiling.  When I was in Montreal, Sylvia told us that we could do that."

At the next dilation session I tried the 45 degree angle ploy and found that it actually worked very well.  After that I kept a book with me and had a good 25 minute stretch during each dilation session where I could read, unhindered.  It certainly made things go faster.

At two to three weeks after surgery the stitches began a long, slow process of unraveling and coming out.  The surgeons use the kind of sutures that dissolve after a while so that folks don't have to make another trip up to Montreal (or even to their own doctors) in order to get stitches removed.  Actually, the first loose stitch I noticed was right in the entrance to the vagina and was loose on one end but still firmly attached on the other.  The reason I noticed it was because the dilators would tug on it as they were being inserted, giving me the impression that a pin was being stuck into my flesh.  A little skillful maneuvering with the mirror and a pair of tweezers convinced me that it wasn't at all ready to come out, so I put up with it for a couple of days until I couldn't take it any more and had Marty snip it for me with a pair of surgical scissors.  She did a good job but was obviously nervous about being in such a sensitive area, and I must admit that seeing a shaky pair of scissors heading for my new vagina would have made me cringe and close my eyes if I hadn't had to hold the flashlight so that she could see what she was doing.

After that, stitches seemed to loosen up and unravel every couple of days for the next month or so.  Some Marty would have to snip for me, others would slide out easily when I gave them a little tug with some tweezers, and still others (I am sure) simply came out without me noticing them while I was doing a pre-dilation soak or while douching.  Phillippa, who I spoke with on the phone at about this time, was experiencing the same thing without the benefit of someone else to do any snipping, and she (tongue-in-cheek, but nevertheless very aptly) described herself as feeling like the bride of Frankenstein.

Family members were the first to come visit me, my mother and my sister, Mary, showing up about four days after I arrived at Marty's house.  Other family members and friends all came around to visit a bit and make sure I was really OK.  I sensed, however, that my parents were still rather concerned, so soon after Thanksgiving (after being at Marty's house for five weeks) I moved into their house for a week before the final move back to my place.  I thought that seeing me at close range for a whole week might be enough to settle their minds and convince them that I wasn't just putting on a brave front while I suffered silently.

After a week with my folks, I packed up my things and made the move back home.  Once back, I gave myself yet another week off from work and used the time to settle back in, reorganize my office space, catch up on correspondence, and generally get my mind and body used to the idea of being active again on a daily basis.

For the previous five weeks I had been dilating four times a day, and I could do that when I wasn't working, but it was pretty obvious that a four-times-a-day schedule was just not going to be easily possible (or even likely) once I was back at work at even the reduced six-hours-per-day I was planning on.  So, once I was back home I immediately cut back to three dilation sessions per day.  I figured that I could do one in the morning before leaving for work, one in the afternoon as soon as I got back from work, and a last session before going to bed at night.

The final thing I did before going back to work was to try using the #3 dilator again, and I was pleased to discover that now (eight weeks after originally starting to dilate and a little less than seven weeks after stopping using it) I had almost no problem with it at all!  It was certainly snug, and still is, but allowing my body and muscles to have almost seven weeks to heal, rest, and regain strength seemed to be what was needed, and after that I was able to slowly increase my time with it until, now, I am on a 5-5-25 minute dilation schedule with no pain at all.

At last, on December 14th, ten weeks after I stopped working, I climbed into my truck and headed back into the work force with a new body and a new life to look forward to.

# FREQUENTLY ASKED QUESTIONS

A lot of people have asked me questions about my sex change, and I find that many of them tend to be variations on the same few questions.  So, to try to anticipate some of the things that you might be wondering, here are the most frequently asked questions that I find myself receiving and the answers that I usually end up giving.

Q:  Do you have orgasms?  If you do, what do they feel like?
A:  Yes, I *do* have orgasms.  The first one I had happened about two and a half months after surgery and was a little mini-orgasm. In other words, I knew something had happened that felt pretty good, but it was rather mild and very quick and, try as I might, I just couldn't get it to happen again at that time.  Since then I've learned a bit more about my new body and can often (though not always) produce an orgasm if I want one.  At this time my orgasms come only from clitoral stimulation, not vaginal stimulation.  Whether that will change as I continue to heal and learn more about what works and what doesn't remains to be seen. What does it feel like?  Well, the nerves that are used to create a clitoris are the nerves that were located in the penis and respon-

108

sible for producing a male orgasm, so the actual, superficial, physical sensation is really not too different from what I felt while having male orgasm.  Still, a few things about my orgasms have definitely changed.  It takes much longer to reach an orgasm now than it used to (no more zero-to-orgasm in five minutes or less).  Achieving an orgasm requires much gentler stimulation now than it used to (no more rushing in like a bull in a china shop).  I absolutely have to be "in the mood" for an orgasm (no longer is it *primarily* a physical thing that can be achieved with little or no romantic feeling), and finally, the feeling during climax is now one that I experience throughout my whole torso (whereas before it was experienced pretty much just in the pe-nis).

Q:   What is it like being a woman?
A:   Not surprisingly, this question only comes to me from men. Invariably, what they mean is:
> A.  What is it like to have breasts?  OR
> B.  What is it like to *not* have a penis?  OR
> C.  What is it like to have breasts and not have a penis?

This is what I tell them:

A.   Despite what your fantasies may be, having breasts is *not* some super sensual feeling that allows you to go around all day in a state of sexual arousal.  Maybe 1% of the time, if you're in the right mood, breasts can be very sensual and bring you a lot of pleasure.  Maybe another 1% of the time, if you're *not* in the right mood, or if you happen to accidentally whack them, they can be downright painful.  The other 98% of the time you hardly even notice that they're there because you're just too busy carrying on with daily life.

B.   Not having a penis is an awful lot like not having a third arm ... and we all know what that feels like, don't we?

C.  For me, having breasts and not having a penis is *wonderful!*  It gives me a completeness, and it gives me a sense of self, and it gives me a feeling of comfort within my own skin that I just never had for more than 40 years of my life.  Obviously, changing one's sex is not something that is going to appeal to everyone (it's not even necessarily going to be the right thing for everyone to whom it appeals), but for me it was right, and I have never felt more whole or more happy with myself ... but then, that's what makes me a transsexual.

Q:  Have you noticed any changes in yourself (other than physical) as a result of the surgery?
A:  *Yes!*  Together with a new sense of wholeness and a new sense of comfort within my own skin there has been a corresponding increase in my spiritual strength, in my centeredness, in my conscious awareness of being immovably "home".  And with that strength and that foundation comes the willingness (I would say even the eagerness) to engage the world more fully to see exactly how well it and I can work and play together for our mutual growth and fulfillment.

Q:  Now that you have a female body, will you be having sex with men?
A:  Probably not.  My sexual attraction has always been towards women and that hasn't changed at all as a result of surgery, so I'm expecting that any future intimate partners will be women. Still, there *is* a part of me that is curious, a part that would like to know, just for the sake of knowing, what it's like to have the experience of being a woman who is made love to by a man.  The problem with that is that I can only think of two men in the whole world who I might be willing to explore that experience with, and both of them are married.  I'm not the kind of person to interfere with any couple's relationship, it's just not my style.  And I am definitely *NOT* about to go into a bar and let some stranger pick

me up and take me home!  Because of those things, I expect
that the opportunity to satisfy my curiosity will remain pretty re-
mote for some time.

Q:   Knowing what you now know about the process, would you
choose to do the surgery all over again if for some reason you
had to?
A:   IN A HEARTBEAT !!!!

## WHERE DOES JEAN FEEL THAT SHE FITS IN

One of the things that I find simultaneously interesting and frustrating (and sometimes hurtful) is how people choose to react to me as a transsexual.

Those folks who do not know that I am transsexual simply accept and treat me as a woman (which is how I view myself as well), but the folks who know that I used to be known as a man (and there are many of them because I have made a conscious decision *not* to deny my past) tend to have a variety of different ideas and behaviors towards me, many of them based on their own internal prejudices and lack of understanding about who I am.

What is interesting to me is that those prejudices exist not only among many fundamentalist religious types (who usually consider me to be some kind of homosexual abomination) but also among many fundamentalist feminist types (for whom I am little more than a "mutilated guy").

What frustrates me about both those prejudices (and about many less-strident notions that I've heard) is how they work to deny me my voice and my right to self-identify and self-determine *who* I am and *how* I fit into the world around me.

What is sometimes hurtful is the often blatant rejection I receive from folks who I can often identify with and with whom I would love to explore friendships.  I am, after all, both deeply spiritual *and* a woman.

So, for the record, I'd like to exercise my voice and share my thoughts on what I think transsexual existence *is* and how I perceive myself fitting into the scheme of things.  Please remember that these are *my* thoughts, *my* feelings, and that they are not shared by all transsexuals.

First of all, I **am** a woman, and I have been a woman since my earliest childhood concept of self-identity.  Whatever other people may have thought of me, whatever life I was encouraged to lead by society, whatever lies I was expected to tell people so that they would feel comfortable dealing with me, my heart and my mind have always been woman-identified.

I wish I could say that I am a woman just like most other women, but if I did that I would be lying to myself just as I lied to the world.  I was never allowed a young girlhood.  I was never allowed a young womanhood.  I came into my completeness middle-aged.  I am a transsexual woman.

I cannot stop you from believing that the word "transsexual" modifies my womanhood enough to destroy it, if that is what you want to believe.  But if that is what you believe, I cannot agree with you.

If that is what you believe, I cannot agree with you because if who we are as human beings is so irrevocably tied to the physical bodies we are born with, and so little dependent on our hearts and spirits, then how can any of us hope to rise above the animal part of our natures and truly soar into the celestial?

In other cultures and in other times, the transsexual people were revered.  They were called twin-spirits; they became the spiritual guides for the community; they acted as mediators; they cared for the orphans.  It was understood that they had the spirit, mind, and heart of one sex, tempered with the knowledge and experience of the other, and that depth of character was re-spected.

In a world where the pursuit of diversity threatens to obscure our memory that we are all *ONE*, transsexuals, by their very existence, stand as a silent testimony from God that even such seemingly diverse and polarized aspects of life as sex (male and female) can become one and live in harmony.  I am a woman who has lived as a man.  I am a transsexual woman ... that is my particular woman-strength.

The transsexual path is *not* for everyone to follow, but it *is* for everyone to learn from.  That learning, however, cannot take place unless there is first acceptance.  Those who deny the womanhood of transsexual women (and the manhood of transsexual men) deny themselves an opportunity for spiritual growth.

I no longer apologize for being who I am.  I no longer hide to protect those with weak sensitivities.  I no longer hand over my power to shallow people of any spiritual or political leaning.  If we, all of us, transgendered and non-transgendered alike, are not *ONE*, then we are not anything.

That is who I am.  That is where I come from.  That is what I think.  My heart belongs to all of you ... you have only to accept it.


**THE END**

Made in the USA
San Bernardino, CA
27 July 2014